Disorders of Language Development

Edited by Pasquale J. Accardo, M.D.,
Brian T. Rogers, M.D., and
Arnold J. Capute, M.D.

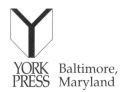

YORK Baltimore,
PRESS Maryland

Volume 6 of the York Spectrum Monographs
A Series based on the Spectrum of Developmental Disabilities Course
sponsored by the Kennedy Fellows Association

This book was manufactured in the United States of America.

Typography by Type Shoppe II Productions, Ltd.
Printing and binding by Data Reproductions Corporation
Cover design by Joseph Dieter, Jr.

Library of Congress Cataloging-In-Publication Data
Disorders of language development / edited by Pasquale J. Accardo, Brian T. Rogers,
and Arnold J. Capute
        p. cm.
    Includes bibliographical references and index.
    ISBN 0-912752-71-8 (pbk.)
      1. Language disorders in children. 2. Child development deviations. 3. Otitis media in
    children--Complications. 4. Children--Language. I. Accardo, Pasquale J. II. Rogers,
    Brian T. III. Capute, Arnold J., 1923.

RJ496.L35 D576 2002
618.92'855--dc21   2002034319

Contents

Contributors

Pasquale J. Accardo, M.D.
Children's Hospital
2924 Brook Road
Richmond, Virginia 23220-1298
and
VCUHS
307 College Street
Randolph Minor Hall
5th Floor, Box 980506
Richmond, Virginia 23298
E-Mail: paccardo@chva.org

Lyn Balsamo, M.A.
Children's Medical Center
111 Michigan Avenue, N.W.
Washington, DC 20010

Joseph H. Beitchman, M.D.
Division of Child Psychiatry
University of Toronto
Hospital for Sick Children, and
Centre for Addiction and Mental
    Health, Clarke Division
Toronto, Ontario
Canada

William Davis Gaillard, M.D.
Children's National Medical
    Center
111 Michigan Avenue, N.W.
Washington, DC 20010
and
Clinical Epilepsy Section
NINDS
National Institutes of Health
Bethesda, Maryland
E-Mail: gaillardw@ninds.nih.gov

Betty Hart, Ph.D.
The University of Kansas
Schiefelbusch Institute for Life
    Span Studies
1052 Dole Human Development
    Center
Lawrence, Kansas 66045
E-Mail:
    schroede@kuhub.cc.ukans.edu

Carla J. Johnson, Ph.D.
Department of Speech-Language
    Pathology
Faculty of Medicine
University of Toronto
Tanz Neuroscience Building
6 Queen's Park Crescent West
Toronto, Ontario M5S 3H2
Canada

Mary L. O'Connor Leppert, M.D.
Johns Hopkins University School of
    Medicine
Kennedy Krieger Institute
Baltimore, Maryland

Andrea S. McDuffie, M.S.,
    CCC-SLP
Department of Special Education
Vanderbilt University
Nashville, Tennessee 37215

Robert J. Ruben, M.D., FACS, FAAP
The University Hospital for the Albert Einstein College of Medicine
3400 Bainbridge Avenue
3rd Floor, Montefiore MC
Bronx, New York 10467-2490
E-Mail: ruben@aecom.yu.edu

Charles T. Snowdon, Ph.D.
Department of Psychology
University of Wisconsin-Madison
W.J. Brogden Psychology Building
1202 West Johnson Street
Mdison, Wisconsin 53706-1696
E-Mail:
    snowdon@facstaff.wisc.edu

Elin T. Thordardottir, Ph.D.
School of Communication Sciences and Disorders
McGill University
Montreal, Quebec
Canada

Susan Ellis Weismer, Ph.D.
Department of Communicative Disorders
Waisman Center
University of Wisconsin-Madison
1500 Highland Avenue
Madison, Wisconsin 53705-2280

Ben Xu, Ph.D.
Clinical Epilepsy Section
NINDS
National Institutes of Health
Bethesda, Maryland

Paul J. Yoder, Ph.D.
Vanderbilt University
Peabody Box 328
Nashville, Tennessee 37215
E-Mail:
    paul.yoder@vanderbilt.edu

Christine Yoshinaga-Itano, Ph.D.
University of Colorado-Boulder
Department of Speech, Language & Hearing Sciences
UCB 409
Boulder, Colorado 80309-0409
E-Mail:
    Christie.Yoshi@colorado.edu

Preface

It is difficult, but not impossible, to overestimate the importance of language to children's development. While a person with no spoken language was in the past referred to as "dumb," the same term was also used to characterize someone with cognitive limitations. Peculiarly, despite the overwhelming importance assigned to language along with the availability of effective intervention strategies, language delays and language disorders in children tend to be diagnosed rather later than either possible or optimal.

Interestingly children learn language in the opposite sequence to which it (and reading) is taught to them. Very young infants will respond positively to the rhythm of spoken sentences (of any language) and negatively to fragmented pieces of the same sentences. Young children will vocalize strings of syllables (jargon) before they begin to connect words in sentences. It is as if they are employing a top-down approach in their first encounters with the spoken word. In contrast many adults will teach children to speak and read individual words before attempting sentences. A parallel phenomenon is the adult who first encounters speakers of a foreign language and perceives that they seem to be speaking their sentences in single long polysyllabic words. The young child has been there. If children acquire language in the reverse order from that which adults use to teach language, it is not surprising that much of our practice and understanding of language disorders in children remains backward.

The importance of early language development as a marker for both specific language problems and for other developmental problems has been increasingly emphasized in pediatrics for the past quarter of a century. Dr. Arnold Capute at Johns Hopkins developed the Clinical and Linguistic Milestone Scale (CLAMS) to help pediatricians assess both expressive and receptive language in infants and young children. He supplemented this instrument with the Clinical Adaptive Test (CAT) to further help differentiate specific language disorders from generalized cognitive impairment and autistic spectrum disorders. That history of special interest in the pediatric approach to early language disorders provided the background to the 2001 Spectrum of Developmental Disabilities course program from which the following chapters have extracted the highpoints.

Pasquale Accardo, M.D.
Richmond, Virginia

Part • I

The Evolution of Language

Chapter • 1

Primate Communication and Language Development

Charles T. Snowdon

Speech and language are uniquely human. Nothing that animals can do approaches the complexity of our vocabulary, our grammar, our ability to express concepts and ideas—both concrete and abstract—our playfulness in punning, and our creativity as we create new words such as "Xerox" and "fax," or to express our love for one another in poetry, to say nothing of our constant talking about language. Even the chimpanzees, gorillas, and other apes that have had years of training to use sign language or symbols on computer keyboards never go much beyond the abilities of a three- or four-year-old child. So why am I writing a chapter about primate communication in a book on *Disorders of Language Development*?

I think there are two important reasons for the relevance of research on primate communication to understanding developmental disorders in language. First, I believe that language did not emerge suddenly in our pre-historic ancestors, but rather language has emerged from and is built upon the abilities of species that preceded humans. That is, language has evolved. Second, we are faced with several competing theories about language and speech development. Is language an instinct that develops normally with minimum effort from caregivers or is language an emergent property from close social interactions between caregivers and infants? It is almost impossible to evaluate these theories based on research with human infants. The understanding of developmental processes can be assisted by looking at developmental processes in closely related species with variation in the types of social interactions in development. In this chapter I will argue for the importance of quality social interactions in language development.

LANGUAGE HAS EVOLVED

Nearly 30 years ago, the linguist Charles Hockett (1963) described 18 features of spoken language. Many of the features relate to aspects of vocal communication that are common to all animals that vocalize, but some of the more interesting features are semanticity (the association of signals with states, objects, or events), arbitrariness (signals do not resemble the event or object they refer to), and discreteness (signals are individual and do not intergrade). These features are found in vervet monkeys that live on the African savannah. Vervet monkeys have separate alarm calls toward each of their major predators: eagles, snakes, and leopards. Playbacks of each of these calls leads to different responses, appropriate to coping with the predator designated by the call (Cheney and Seyfarth 1990). Others of Hockett's features are: Tradition (transmitting signals through teaching or learning) seen in many birds where songs are learned from older adults, and in dolphins and bats where animals with close social relationships develop similar calls; Displacement (referring to objects or events remote in space or time) seen in the waggle dance of honey bees which communicates the direction and distance to nectar sources; Openness (forming new signals through blending and transforming) seen in both chimpanzees and parrots that have been trained by humans (for example, the parrot, Alex, blends the previously acquired words of "banana" and "cherry" into "bannery" on first encountering an apple); Syntax (predictable order or sequencing of signals) found in birds like chickadees and some monkeys (and chickadees even display a simple form of generative grammar (Hailman, Ficken, and Ficken 1985); Prevarication (conscious lying or deceit) seen in chimpanzees; Learnability (speakers of one language learning other languages) seen in examples of primates of one species responding to alarm calls of other species, birds, or other mammals (for example, vervet monkeys on the African savannah learn to respond to alarm calls given by superb starlings, Hauser 1988); and Duality of Patterning (combining different sounds into words or words into phrases with the differing orders of similar elements having different meanings) seen in responses to novel sequences in both dolphins and chimpanzees trained in a language analogue (see Snowdon 1999, 2001 for specific details). Only one of Hockett's features of language is not yet seen in nonhuman species: Reflexiveness (the ability to communicate about communicating). Although most of Hockett's design features can be found in some nonhuman species, no single nonhuman species has all of the design features that Hockett proposed.

In addition, several studies (see Kluender 1994 and Kuhl 1987 for reviews) have found that a variety of nonhuman species ranging from Japanese quail to chinchillas to macaques perceive human speech sounds in a human-like way. If nonhuman species as far distant as quail perceive human speech sounds as humans do, then the origins of perception of speech must be quite ancient. All of these results taken together suggest that human language has its origins from the communication systems of other species. That is, rather than create an entirely new communication system from scratch, our ancestors built language ability upon traits found in other species. This makes sense for it is much easier to build upon a pre-existing foundation of perceptual, motor, and cognitive skills than to develop a complex skill from no precursors. Thus, language has evolved from more primitive abilities of other species.

HOW DID LANGUAGE BECOME SO COMPLEX?

It is not enough to consider what components of language might have emerged from our nonhuman ancestors, but we must also ask what has led to the enormous eruption of complexity seen in human languages. The complexity of language is all the more striking given the relative simplicity of vocal communication in the great apes, our closest relatives. John Mitani, who has studied communication in wild apes more than anyone else, has reported that there are relatively few discretely different signals in apes, and no evidence of the type of semantic communication about objects in the environment seen in vervet monkeys and other species (Mitani 1996). Harcourt and Stewart (2001) claim that mountain gorillas have the most complex vocal communication of all apes, yet there are only 12 different calls. When I visited mountain gorillas at the famous Karisoke Research Center in Rwanda many years ago, I was impressed with how quiet the mountain gorillas were compared with the forest monkeys that I study. So if great apes are relatively silent and have an impoverished vocal repertoire compared with forest monkeys (or even birds), how have humans become such a chattering species?

Apes have very expressive facial expressions and use gestures extensively (van Hooff 1972; Snowdon 2002), which might be complex enough for their social needs (and which is why the earliest successful attempts to teach some aspects of language to apes used American Sign

Language). We humans have retained the complexity of facial expression and gestures seen in apes, but have added vocal complexity as well.

Vocal communication has several advantages. Humans and apes have highly overlapping visual fields that give us great binocular depth perception, but limit our ability to see things to our sides or behind us. We miss more than half of our visual world, but vocalizations can be heard from every direction. Furthermore, using vocalizations, we can communicate in the dark, and in deep forests, and we can keep our hands free for carrying tools, weapons, or other material goods. Thus, those of our ancestors who increased the complexity and use of vocal communication would have benefitted compared to those who did not. The expansion of vocalizations might have started by referring to predators and food types (as seen in many monkeys and even chickens!). But then if vocalizations could be used as well to make requests or coordinate social activities, an expansion of these calls would have occurred very rapidly and benefitted those with these increased language abilities. Those of our ancestors who could communicate more effectively about the location of food, shelter, and predators and who could manage their social interactions more effectively would have greater reproductive success—meaning more surviving offspring, and better choice of mating partners. Thus, communication skills could have evolved rapidly in a way consistent with the rapid expansion of brain size that occurred (Noble and Davidson 1994), eventually resulting in the complex language we know today. Furthermore, it is easy to imagine that those who could readily transfer their communication skills to their infants through teaching would ensure that their children had an advantage later in life. This leads us now to the main focus of this volume: language development and disabilities.

A LANGUAGE INSTINCT?

Because children seem to acquire language so quickly and proficiently across a wide variation in environments, it has become popular to think of language as innate or instinctive. Some writers (e.g., Pinker 1994) have posited an innate Language Acquisition Device, and specific "modules" in the brain dedicated to things like plurals, past tense, passive voice, etc. How we interpret the notion of innateness, or instinct, is crucial for all of those involved in treating developmental disorders of language. If speech and language are completely controlled by biological processes of development, then there is little to be gained by therapeutic intervention. On the other hand, if speech and language have a biological basis that requires some learning and experience for full expression, then therapeutic intervention does become important.

Clearly there is a biological basis for language. At the very minimum, speech requires a vocal tract with appropriate articulators in order to produce sounds of language, as well as a brain with the potential to control the articulators and to decode the sounds of language. But the necessity for these biological supports for speech does not mean that there is no role for experience or social interaction in language and speech development. As an analogy consider driving a car. Most humans are born with the arms, legs, eyesight, and brain capacity to be able to drive a car, but most of us require some instruction and lots of practice in order to drive a car well. (We also must be able to solve simultaneous differential equations in order to effectively decelerate and turn a corner, but few of us understand the formal solutions of such equations.) The fact that a biological basis for driving exists does not mean that teaching, learning, and practicing are not important too.

Several arguments have been made in favor of a language instinct. One is that there are universals across all languages and over development. Although there are some universals (Jakobsen and Halle 1956), many appear to me to be trivial: All languages use stop consonants and most use three places of articulation represented by /ba/, /da/, and /ga/. Most languages use the vowels [I], [a], and [u], vowels that chimpanzees cannot produce. However, despite these universals, there is great phonetic diversity. The UCLA Phonological Segment Database (Maddieson 1984) describes 558 consonants, 260 vowels, and 51 diphthongs, with great variability in the number of phonemes within a language (from 11 phonemes in Rotaka and Mura to 141 phonemes in !Xu). This great variability in phonemes among languages suggests that great flexibility is required in learning to speak. Infants begin babbling using a wide array of phonemes and can perceive phonetic contrasts not found in their native language, but by 10 to 12 months of age there is a selective loss of perceptual contrasts not needed for the infant's native language (Werker and Teas 1984), and infants at this age recognize the intonation contours of their native language (Hirsch-Pasek et al. 1987) and produce the sounds of their native language in babbling (Boysson-Bardies, Sagart, and Durand 1984).

Another argument has been for universals in development of grammar. However, Bates and Marchman (1988) have argued that most of the studies favoring universals in development of grammar have focused mainly on the sequence of development in English speaking children. When one looks at languages with different grammatical emphases such as Turkish, Russian, and Italian, along with English, there are clear differences depending on the importance within each language of word order, case endings, complexity of verb endings, and gender. Turkish children, where case endings are more important than word order, master case endings early, whereas English children master word order early. Three-year-old Italian children use relative clauses much more frequently than English children. Bates and Marchman (1988) argue that children appear to learn earliest the aspects of grammar most important in their own language rather than following a universal trajectory. Even within English, they argue, the onset of words, phrases, and acquiring negative or passive forms is highly variable across individuals. Children with brain damage in areas thought to be critical to language production or comprehension can recover language skills with appropriate training so that they have normal or near normal levels of language ability as adults. Biological markers of brain development do not appear to be correlated with emergence of specific capacities for speech or grammar, and there is bi-directionality between brain growth and behavior with complex learning in adults leading to increased growth in both number of nerve cells and the number of synapses on each cell (see Bates et al. in press for a review).

Another argument is that there are critical periods in language development, implying that after a certain age there is a permanent disability of language acquisition. However, evidence of critical periods in humans is difficult to obtain. Many case examples relate to children who were socially isolated by abusive parents. What is the cause of the language deficits they display? Lack of exposure to others? Malnutrition? Cumulative effects of chronic abuse? Severe brain damage or retardation in infancy that led the parents to isolate them? We really cannot distinguish among these possibilities, and one might argue that any child who has been socially isolated is likely to experience multiple disorders. Even studies of songbirds that first established the idea of critical periods in vocal development (Marler 1970) are now tempered by evidence that housing birds with social companions can extend the period for song development, and even lead to the development of song of a different species if the social companion is from a different species (Baptista and Gaunt 1997).

Adults can learn second languages, although few of us show the same proficiency as we do with our native languages (Johnson and Newport 1989). However, there is a remarkable example from an isolated part of the Amazon at the border between Brazil and Colombia. Here an indigenous population uses 25 different languages from 4 different language families. Because marriage occurs outside of one's own group, an infant is likely to grow up learning her father's and her mother's languages, and when she marries, the languages of her spouse and each of her in-laws. It is claimed that adults value proficiency in multiple languages although actual details of proficiency are not available (Sorenson 1967). This suggests that with sufficient motivation, adults might learn several additional languages to reasonable proficiency. Note that the motivation here is social, communicating competently with those having close social relationships, a point that I will return to later.

The quality of social relationships also affects language acquisition. Jouanjean-l'Antoene (1997) reported on a pair of twins whose language development she studied intensively from 11 months to 23 months. Each twin had a preferred parent for social interactions: one interacted most with the mother who remained in the home, the other with her father who was absent for a long period early in the second year. Although both parents directed equal amounts of language to each child, there was more reciprocity within the preferred dyad. Although both twins vocalized at equal rates with each parent, the mother imitated and expanded on vocalizations much more with her preferred twin, and that twin produced a higher proportion of linguistic utterances than her sister.

Several studies suggest that children who are neglected have severe delays in language development; however, children who have been physically abused, or both neglected and abused, show normal language development (Allen and Oliver 1982; Fox, Long, and Langlois 1988; Culp et al. 1991). Locke and Snow (1997) argue that language emerges from close social interactions between caregivers and infants, and they further hypothesize that abused children may become more strongly bonded to their caregivers than non-abused infants, paradoxically assisting the abused child to acquire language skills as readily as a nonabused child. In contrast, the neglected child is missing the social interactions that are essential for language learning.

Finally, learning about language might occur very rapidly, so rapidly that it might not be easy to observe under normal conditions. Saffran, Aslin and Newport (1996) described a new type of learning process, statistical learning. They presented 8-month-old infants with a two-minute sequence of nonsense syllables. However, some triads of syllables occurred together in the same order 70% of the time, others 50% of the time, and others did not occur together. After hearing the two-minute stimulus sequence, the infants were tested in a head turning paradigm, and showed habituation to the triads that had occurred together 50% or 70%, but treated as novel sequences that had occurred together only once. Saffran et al. (1996) argue that the frequently co-occurring nonsense syllables are analogous to words and suggest that infants are able to use statistical learning to extract meaningful acoustic patterns from a seemingly undifferentiated stream of acoustic information, and they can do so quickly. This type of learning is not limited to speech sounds but is effective in learning sequences of tones as well (Saffran et al. 1999) Statistical learning provides a mechanism for understanding how infants can appear to acquire language skills so quickly, but without invoking some innate and unknown Language Acquisition Device.

NONHUMAN ANIMAL MODELS

There have been three difficulties in considering nonhuman animal models for understanding the development of language. First, no animals display anything approximating the complexity of human languages, but as I argued earlier, many of the characteristics of language can be seen in some nonhuman species. Thus, nonhuman animals might be useful models for certain aspects of language. Second, the great apes, our closest relatives, do not vocalize often nor, from what we know at present, do they appear to have complex vocalizations. This creates a problem if we think of evolutionary processes in a traditional way, with only those species most closely related to humans being of interest. However, although great apes share many of our genes in common, they have evolved very different social organizations. Gorillas live in harem groups with one or two males having control over several females. Orangutans are generally solitary with little permanent social organization beyond a mother and her offspring. Chimpanzees live in continuously shifting subgroups within a larger community with only temporary relationships between males and females. In contrast, in most modern human cultures the family is the unit of social organization. If we agree with Locke and Snow (1997) that close social interactions between caregivers and infants are fundamental to language development, then our best nonhuman models might be species that also live in families.

Third, there has been, until recently, little evidence of vocal development in nonhuman primates. Seyfarth and Cheney (1997) in a thorough review of vocal development distinguish between production, usage, and comprehension. They found considerable evidence that primates can learn to understand calls of their own and other species, but there was much less evidence of plasticity in the use of calls in appropriate contexts, although some learning appeared. There was least evidence for learning in producing calls. This might be expected in part, given the limitations imposed on production by the structure of the vocal tract and articulatory structures. However, Seyfarth and Cheney also noted that studies in the last decade or so had provided more evidence of what they called "modification within constraints."

My own research on primate vocal development has concentrated on cotton-top tamarins and pygmy marmosets. Both of these species are from South America and are considered, along with other marmosets and tamarins, to be cooperative breeders. Unlike other nonhuman primates, these monkeys live in small family groups, where there is typically only one breeding male and one breeding female. However, all group members contribute to the successful rearing of infants with mothers nursing infants, but fathers and older siblings doing most of the carrying and care taking throughout the day. These monkeys live in heavily forested areas where vocal communication is much more useful than gesturing or other visual signals. These monkeys have among the largest vocal repertoires of any primates (35 different vocalizations in cotton-top tamarins (Cleveland and Snowdon 1982), 25 different vocalizations in pygmy marmosets (Pola and Snowdon 1975). Therefore, these monkeys have a social organization more similar to humans than the great apes, and they have a much more complex vocal repertoire than the great apes. Let us now look at some of the developmental processes we have studied in these species.

Babbling is characteristic of all human infants, but an equivalent phenomenon is rarely seen in other species. We have found that pygmy marmoset infants produce long streams of vocalizations that we have termed "pygmy marmoset babbling" (Elowson, Snowdon, and Lazaro-Perea 1998). These complex vocalizations share many features with human babbling. During these complex vocal sequences, the infant marmosets produce about 60% of the call types used by adults and most of the calls are clearly recognizable from the adult repertoire (as in the canonical babbling of infants). The calls are often repeated in sequences of two-four repetitions of the same call type (similar to reduplicative babbling in infants). The sequence of calls produced bears little resemblance to the infant's ongoing behavior. Calls that in adults would communicate threat are juxtaposed with those given by adults in calm social interactions within a group, then with those used in feeding, and those used in response to spotting a predator. That is, for the infants there is no semantic (or at least adult semantic) structure in the calls. This pygmy marmoset babbling also leads to increased social interactions with other family members. Infants are more often with other group members or more likely to approach or be approached by family members when they are babbling than when they are not. This babbling behavior is not an artifact of captivity, since we have also heard it in pygmy marmosets living in the western Amazon, and we have also observed similar vocal behavior in a related species, the common marmoset, in its habitat in Northeast Brazil. The major concentration of babbling occurs in the early weeks of life beginning before weaning and declining as the infants get older.

We find that the rate of babbling decreases, but the proportion of adult-like forms of calls increases with age. We also find a more accurate production of adult calls (Snowdon and Elowson 2001). Trill vocalizations are the most commonly used calls of adult pygmy marmosets and were the most frequent call type found in babbling. We looked closely at the structure of trills and found different time courses for achieving control over structure. Trills increased to adult duration in the first five months, whereas other components of trill structure did not appear to be under precise vocal control until adulthood. We also found that the amount of change in trill structure among individual monkeys over the first five months was directly related to the amount and diversity of babbling. Infants who vocalized more and with greater diversity showed the fastest progression toward adult structure in the first five months, although when all animals were tested as adults (at three years of age) there was little variation in trill structure. Therefore, although there were different developmental trajectories produced as a function of amount of babbling in infancy, all monkeys eventually acquired adult structure.

Pygmy marmosets also display vocal plasticity as adults. Different populations of pygmy marmosets in the Amazon, separated by 100 km, have different forms of some of their calls (de la Torre 1999). This is the first natural evidence of dialects among wild monkeys. Whether these dialects are due to genetic differences between the two populations or to learning is unclear. However, pygmy marmosets do alter vocal structure as adults. In one study, we studied the vocalizations of our own colony and of another colony we received from another institution while the latter group was in quarantine. We recorded trills from individuals in each of the two colonies before and after we began to house all monkeys in the same large colony room. Although the colonies were still housed in separate family groups, all individuals demonstrated changes in trill structure within 6 weeks of putting the two colonies in the same room (Elowson and Snowdon 1994). Later we studied the trills of individual marmosets before and after pairing with an unfamiliar monkey. In the three pairs where the individual trill structure varied before pairing, all converged on a single form of trill, going from "his" call and "her" call to "their" call. Three years later the same pairs still had similar trill structure (Snowdon and Elowson 1999).

Adult pygmy marmosets show plasticity in trill structures, and changes in social environment or social partners appear to be a major variable leading to vocal change. In humans there is evidence of vocal accommodation, changes in our pronunciation or usage of language as we join new social groups. This alteration in vocal structure serves as a "social badge" that acknowledges that a change in social group membership has occurred and that we accept our new social role.

All of the changes in vocal structure we found in adult pygmy marmosets were subtle modifications to existing call structure. That is, pygmy marmosets are not learning completely new vocalizations outside of the species repertoire, but within the physical constraints of their body size and vocal apparatus, they can change subtle aspects of call structure, much as humans can learn a new dialect or a second language.

The cotton-top tamarin has an elaborate set of vocalizations. We have found 8 variants of short, high-pitched, frequency-modulated calls that we have labeled as chirps. Each of these 8 variants is used in a particular context: one is associated with mobbing a threatening stimulus, one leads to silence and immobility in response to sudden loud noises, two are associated with feeding—one as animals approach food, and the other after food is selected, another is given in response to hearing calls of an unfamiliar group, and another is given in calm intragroup settings. We can do a distinctive features analysis of the 8 chirps and separate each chirp on the basis of two or three acoustic features (Cleveland and Snowdon 1982). The monkeys themselves distinguish among the chirp types. We selected the acoustically most similar forms of chirps and played them back to several groups of tamarins through hidden speakers. Although the chirps were less than $1/20$ of a second in duration, after hearing just two chirps, the monkeys responded differently, and appropriately, to each type of chirp (Bauers and Snowdon 1990).

We developed several different experimental manipulations, each designed to elicit one type of chirp, and tested several family groups with each manipulation. Adults responded to each type of experimental setting with the appropriate chirp type, and we saw no mixing of chirp types across different contexts (Castro and Snowdon 2000). How do infant tamarins develop competence in the production and use of chirps? According to earlier studies of primate vocal development where calls appeared to be fully formed at birth, a young tamarin when presented with each of the situations, which would elicit a specific chirp type in adults, should respond with the appropriate chirp. However, this did not occur. First, we found little evidence of adult chirp types in infants up to 5 months of age (the equivalent of a toddler). Instead infants used a series of chirps that matched few of the specific features of the adult chirps. These "prototype" chirps were used in all situations (Castro and Snowdon 2000). On some occasions, an infant would give an appropriate chirp in response to an experimental test, but there was great variation with most infants giving some of the chirps and few giving others. In no case did the same infant give each of the appropriate chirp types in our experiment. Furthermore, once an infant produced a chirp in an appropriate context, the probability of producing the chirp again in a subsequent test was less than 25% (Castro and Snowdon 2000). Thus, tamarin infants do not appear to have an "instinct" for how to produce or how to use their vocalizations.

There was one exception to the pattern I have described. The D-Chirp, which is given by adults in response to feeding on a preferred food, was used on more than 40% of subsequent trials by infant tamarins once they had given it. Adult cotton-top tamarins share food with infants beginning at about 6 weeks of age. Typically a male picks up a piece of food and holds it out to an infant while simultaneously producing a series of D-chirp calls. In food-sharing with infants, the adults produce a louder and much longer series of these chirps than they do when feeding on their own, and in about 15% of the tests we did, other group members would orient toward the adult and infant and give series of D-chirp vocalizations themselves (Roush and Snowdon 2001). Only when the adult vocalizes is an infant successful in obtaining food. Tamarins that are involved in food sharing earlier in life show earlier production of the D-chirp and of independent feeding. This type of food sharing has been seen in other species of marmosets and tamarins, with adults more likely to share highly preferred foods, foods that are difficult to obtain, and foods that are familiar to adults, but unfamiliar to the infants (Rapaport 1999). Thus food sharing, and the accompanying production of food-associated calls (D-chirps) create a context for learning about food and about the vocalizations appropriate for feeding. Food sharing appears to be a form of active teaching of infants about food.

It is possible that food vocalizations are still innate, requiring appropriate stimulation to elicit the calls, but with no subsequent developmental modification. We studied several infants, juveniles, and subadults ranging in age from 4 to 28 months of age (puberty occurs at about 18 months). We found evidence of over-generalization: young monkeys would give food vocalizations to small non-food toys, and we found that many of the calls produced in response to food were clearly similar to adult calls, but more variable, outside the range of adult variation. In addition, young tamarins produced many other vocalizations not observed in adults in a feeding context. To our surprise both the variability in D-chirp production, the production of other calls, and the over-generalization of usage did not change with increasing age nor change after puberty (Roush and Snowdon 1994).

As cooperative breeders, tamarins typically have only one breeding adult of each sex while the other group members are reproductively inhibited. We hypothesized that juvenile and subadult monkeys might benefit by communication of their subordinate social status through continued "baby-talk." To test this hypothesis we tested subadults living in their family groups and again after they had been paired with a new mate and housed apart from their families. There was a rapid change in behavior on food trials with newly paired adults giving only food associated calls without the other vocal types, and producing chirps within the range of adult variation (Roush and Snowdon 1999). Thus social stimuli from family members are not only important in developing normal vocal development, but can also inhibit vocal development when it is to the advantage of the young to communicate subordinate status. We also find that adult pygmy marmosets learn to use babbling as a way to get access to resources and to indicate subordinate status during aggressive interactions.

PRIMATE COMMUNICATION AND LANGUAGE DISORDERS

These studies of pygmy marmosets and cotton-top tamarins suggest that both the adult-type production and adult-appropriate use of communication signals are strongly influenced by social interactions within families. Although I have not provided direct evidence of learning, there is clearly plasticity or modifiability in the communication of at least these primates. If these primates display plasticity and flexibility in response to social interactions, then we need to at least entertain the hypothesis that similar social variables affect human language development as well.

One of the remarkable components of vocal development in both pygmy marmosets and cotton-top tamarins is the responsiveness of caretakers to infant vocalizations, and creating contexts for learning to occur. In no other group of nonhuman primates do we find food sharing that involves an adult offering food to an infant while simultaneously emphasizing the vocalizations used in feeding. Remarkably, other group members often orient to the food sharing adult and infant and vocalize as well. Food sharing creates a joint attention between an adult and infant that draws the infant's attention to food and to appropriate vocalizations.

In human infants, the emergence of joint attention at about 9 to 10 months is hypothesized to be a critical stage in the infant's ability to imitate both sounds and actions (Tomasello 1999) and necessary for the development of cognitive and linguistic complexity. In each of the successful studies where scientists have trained nonhuman animals to use language, a key component is the development of joint attention between the scientist and the animal being trained (for African gray parrots, Pepperberg 1999; for chimpanzees, Savage-Rumbaugh and Levin 1994). This even applies to robots! Steels and Kaplan (2001) have shown that a robotic dog, AIBO, learns words only through joint attention. In each case, the physical presence of a social companion who directs the attention of an infant, a parrot, a chimpanzee, or a robot to objects and associated names is necessary. Word acquisition with appropriate reference is not successful through auditory or video playbacks alone or even when a social companion is present but not interacting with the tutee. If language acquisition were innate, then this intensive interaction between adults and infants should not be necessary. But the critical importance of joint attention in the nonhuman examples (both animal and robot) attests to the probable critical importance in human infants too.

What does all of this mean for treating developmental disorders of language? First, and most important, a therapist can play an important and critical role. If one accepts the "Language Instinct" hypothesis, then there would be little, if any, role for a therapist, but intervention should make a difference according to the view I've presented. Second, intervention and treatment should work best in the context of a family. Human infants and young marmosets and tamarins grow up in families, and the primary social relationships that are established within families are likely to be the ones most effective in producing change. So I suggest that therapists should make use of families, training family members to assist in treatment. Third, development of joint attention between the child and both the therapist and family members should be important in developing effective treatment.

KEY POINTS

Speech and language are uniquely human, but have evolved from communication systems in nonhuman species.

Many "design features" of language can be observed in other species, but no single nonhuman species displays all the features of language.

Although there is a clear biological basis for language and language development, there is little objective evidence for "Innate Language Acquisition Devices" or a "Language Instinct."

There are few significant universals in language or its development suggesting that rapid individual learning within the context of a social group or culture is a more parsimonious explanation of language development.

Our closest relatives, the great apes, use elaborate gestural signals, but have relatively impoverished vocal communication. They also live in social groups much different from the family organization of many human societies.

In contrast, family-living marmosets and tamarins display many parallels to human vocal development including vocal practice through babbling, creating a context for teaching about food and appropriate calls, and the ability to alter vocal structure even as adults in response to social changes.

Joint attention involving an infant and a strong social partner is a key feature in language and cognitive development in human and tamarin infants, in studies training parrots or chimpanzees to acquire aspects of language, and even in robots.

These results taken together argue strongly for an important role of therapists working within the family context to address developmental disorders of speech and language.

ACKNOWLEDGMENTS

Supported by USPHS Grant MH 29775 and funds from the University of Wisconsin Graduate School Research Committee.

REFERENCES

Allen, R. E., and Oliver, J. M. 1982. The effect of child maltreatment on language development. *Child Abuse and Neglect* 6:299–305.

Baptista, L. F., and Gaunt, S. L. L. 1997. Social interaction and vocal development in birds. In *Social Influences on Vocal Development*, eds. C. T. Snowdon and M. Hausberger. Cambridge: Cambridge University Press.

Bates, E., and Marchman, V. 1988. What is and is not universal in language acquisition. In *Language Communication and the Brain*, ed. F. Plum. New York: Raven Press.

Bates, E., Thal, D., Finlay, B., and Clancy, B. In press. Early language development and its neural correlates. In *Handbook of Neuropsychology, Vol. 7 Child Neurology, (2nd edition)*, eds. I. Rapin and S. Segalowitz. Amsterdam: Elsevier.

Bauers, K. A., and Snowdon, C. T. 1990. Discrimination of chirp variants in the cotton-top tamarin. *American Journal of Primatology* 21:53–60.

Boysson-Bardies, B., Sagart, L., and Durand, C. 1984. Discernible differences in the babbling of infants according to target language. *Journal of Child Language* 11:1–15.

Castro, N. A., and Snowdon, C. T. 2000. Development of vocal responses in infant cotton-top tamarins. *Behaviour* 137:629–46.

Cheney, D. L., and Seyfarth, R. M. 1990. *How Monkeys See the World*. Chicago: University of Chicago Press.

Cleveland, J., and Snowdon, C. T. 1982. The complex vocal repertoire of the adult cotton-top tamarin (*Saguinus oedipus oedipus*). *Zeitschrift fur Tierpsychologie* 58:231–70.

Culp, R. E., Watkins, R. V., Lawrence, H., Letts, D., Kelly, D. J., and Rice, M. L. 1991. Maltreated children's language and speech development: abused, neglected, and abused and neglected. *First Language* 11:377–89.

De la Torre, S. 1999. Environmental correlates of vocal communication of wild pygmy marmosets, *Cebuella pygmaea*. Unpublished Doctoral Dissertation, University of Wisconsin, Madison.

Elowson, A. M., and Snowdon, C. T. 1994. Pygmy marmosets, *Cebuella pyg-maea*, modify vocal structure in response to changed social environment. *Animal Behaviour* 47:1267–77.

Elowson, A. M., Snowdon, C. T., and Lazaro-Perea, C. 1998. Infant "babbling" in a nonhuman primate: Complex vocal sequences with repeated call types. *Behaviour* 135:643–64.

Fox, L., Long, S. H., and Langlois, A. 1988. Patterns of language comprehension deficit in abused and neglected children. *Journal of Speech and Hearing Disorders* 53:239–44.

Hailman, J. P., Ficken, M. S., and Ficken, R. W. 1985. The "chick-a-dee" call of *Parus atricapillus*: A recombinant system of animal communication compared with written English. *Semiotica* 56:191–224.

Harcourt, A. H., and Stewart, K. J. 2001. Vocal relationships of wild mountain gorillas. In *Mountain Gorillas: Three Decades of Research at Karisoke*, eds. M. M. Robbins, P. Sicotte, and K. J. Stewart. Cambridge: Cambridge University Press.

Hauser, M. D. 1988. How vervet monkeys learn to recognize starling alarm calls: The role of experience. *Behaviour* 105:187–201.

Hirsch-Pasek, K., Kemler Nelson, D., Jusczyk, P. W., Cassidy, K., Druss, B., and Kennedy, L. 1987. Clauses are perceptual units for young infants. *Cognition* 26:269–86.

Hockett, C. F. 1963. The problem of universals in language. In *Universals of Language*, ed. J. H. Greenberg. Cambridge, MA: MIT Press.

Van Hooff, J. A. R. A. M. 1972. A comparative approach to the phylogeny of laughter and smiling. In *Nonverbal Communication*, ed. R. A. Hinde. Cambridge: Cambridge University Press.

Jakobson, R., and Halle, M. 1956. *Fundamentals of Language.* s'Gravenhage: Mouton.

Johnson, J. S., and Newport, E. M. 1989. Critical periods in second language learning: the influence of maturational state on the acquisition of English as a second language. *Cognitive Psychology* 21:60–99.

Jouanjean-l'Antoene, A. 1997. Reciprocal interactions and the development of communication and language between parents and children. In *Social Influences on Vocal Development*, eds. C. T. Snowdon and M. Hausberger. Cambridge: Cambridge University Press.

Kluender, K. R. 1994. Speech perception as a tractable problem in cognitive science. In *Handbook of Psycholinguistics*, ed. M. A. Gernsbacher. San Diego: Academic Press.

Kuhl, P. K. 1987. The special mechanisms debate in speech: contributions of tests on animals (and the relation of these tests using non-speech stimuli). In *Categorical Perception*, ed. S. Harnad. Cambridge: Cambridge University Press.

Locke, J. L., and Snow, C. 1997 Social influences in vocal learning in human and nonhuman primates. In *Social Influences on Vocal Development*, eds. C. T. Snowdon and M. Hausberger. Cambridge: Cambridge University Press.

Maddieson, I. 1984. *Patterns of Sound.* Cambridge: Cambridge University Press.

Marler, P. 1970. Birdsong and speech development: Could there be parallels? *American Scientist* 58:669–73.

Mitani, J. C. 1996. Comparative studies of African ape vocal behavior. In *Great Ape Societies*, eds. W. C. McGrew, L. F. Marchant, and T. Nishida. Cambridge: Cambridge University Press.

Noble, W., and Davidson, I. 1994. *Human Evolution, Language and the Mind: A Psychological and Archeological Inquiry.* Cambridge: Cambridge University Press.

Pepperberg, I. M. 1999. *The Alex Studies*. Cambridge MA: Harvard University Press.

Pinker, S. 1994. *The Language Instinct*. New York: William Morrow.

Pola, Y. V., and Snowdon, C. T. 1975. The vocalizations of pygmy marmosets (*Cebuella pygmaea*). *Animal Behaviour* 23:826–42.

Rapaport, L. G. 1999. Provisioning of young in golden lion tamarins (Callithrichidae, *Leontopithecus rosalia*): A test of the information hypothesis. *Ethology* 105:619–36.

Roush, R. S., and Snowdon, C. T. 1994. Ontogeny of food-associated calls in cotton-top tamarins. *Animal Behaviour* 47:263–73.

Roush, R. S., and Snowdon, C. T. 1999. The effects of social status on food-associated calling behaviour in captive cotton-top tamarins. *Animal Behaviour* 58:1299–1305.

Roush, R. S., and Snowdon, C. T. 2001. Food transfers and the development of feeding behavior and food-associated vocalizations in cotton-top tamarins. *Ethology* 107:415–29.

Saffran, J. R., Aslin, R. N., and Newport, E. L. 1996. Statistical learning in 8-month-old infants. *Science* 274:1926–8.

Saffran, J. R., Johnson, E. K., Aslin, R. N., and Newport, E. L. 1999. Statistical learning of tone sequences by human infants and adults. *Cognition* 70:27–52.

Savage-Rumbaugh, E., and Levin, R. 1994. *Kanzi: The Ape on the Brink of Human Mind*. New York: John Wiley.

Seyfarth, R. M., and Cheney, D. L. 1997. Some general features of vocal development in primates. In *Social Influences on Vocal Development*, eds. C. T. Snowdon and M. Hausberger. Cambridge: Cambridge University Press.

Snowdon, C. T. 1999. An empiricist view of language evolution and development. In *The Origins of Language: What Nonhuman Primates Can Tell Us*, ed. B. J. King. Santa Fe: School of American Research Press.

Snowdon, C. T. 2001. From primate communication to human language. In *Tree of Origin*, ed. F. B. M. de Waal. Cambridge, MA: Harvard University Press.

Snowdon, C. T. 2002 Expression of emotion in nonhuman animals. In *Handbook of Affective Science*, eds. R. J. Davidson, K. Scherer and H. H. Goldsmith. New York: Oxford University Press.

Snowdon, C. T., and Elowson, A. M. 1999. Pygmy marmosets modify call structure when paired. *Ethology* 105:893–908.

Snowdon, C. T., and Elowson, A. M. 2001. "Babbling" in pygmy marmosets: Development after infancy. *Behaviour* 138:1235–48.

Sorensen, A. P., Jr. 1967. Multilingualism in the Northwest Amazon. *American Anthropologist* 69:670–85.

Steels, L., and Kaplan, F. 2000. AIBO's first words. The social learning of language and meaning. *Evolution of Communication*, 4:3–32.

Tomasello, M. 1999. *The Cultural Origins of Human Cognition*. Cambridge, MA: Harvard University Press.

Werker, J., and Teas, R. 1984. Cross-language speech perception: Evidence for perceptual reorganization during the first year of life. *Infant Behavior and Development* 7:49–63.

Chapter • 2

Cognition and Language

Susan Ellis Weismer and
Elin T. Thordardottir

There has been considerable interest among psychologists and scholars in a host of related fields in characterizing the nature of the relationship between language and cognition in both typical and atypical cases. Work in this area has focused on constructing theoretical accounts of the link between language and cognitive functioning in adults, as well as explaining developmental patterns observed in infancy and childhood. Historically, the conceptualization of this relationship has ranged from claims that language directs thought, exemplified by the Sapir-Whorfian notion of linguistic determinism, to accounts at the other end of the spectrum that have emphasized the influence of cognition on language, as in the strong form of the cognitive hypothesis based on a Piagetian framework.

Current modularity accounts (Pinker 1994), stemming from earlier claims of highly specialized systems subserving language (Chomsky 1964, 1988; Fodor 1983), assume that linguistic knowledge is encapsulated and largely independent of other cognitive domains. This view can be contrasted with various perspectives that assume an interactionist position, including connectionist and dynamic systems accounts that espouse an emergent view of language acquisition. As noted by MacWhinney (1999), emergent accounts of language development offer an alternative to the long-standing opposition between nativism and empiricism in that emergentism focuses on accounting, in mechanistic terms, for interactions between biological and environmental processes. Within this type of framework, we might expect that the nature of the interplay between language and cognition will shift in a dynamic manner as a function of a child's developmental trajectory.

Various researchers, particularly those seeking support for modularity claims, have been interested in examining ways in which language and cognitive functioning can become disassociated in atypical cases. Within the field of cognitive neuropsychology, adult neurological patients who demonstrate a dissociation between two areas of functioning are studied in order to gain insights into normal cognitive processes. Of particular interest are double dissociations involving patients who demonstrate mirror image patterns of deficits, which are seen as evidence for the notion that these aspects of functioning are logically independent.

This approach has been increasingly applied to developmental disorders as well as to acquired disorders in adults. Two types of developmental language disorders (characterized by uneven profiles) that have been examined within this framework include Williams syndrome and specific language impairment. Children with Williams syndrome (WS) have been characterized as having relatively complex language despite having generally deficient cognitive abilities, whereas children with specific language impairment (SLI) present a profile of poor language skills in the face of normal nonverbal abilities. On the surface, these patterns appear to represent a prototypic double dissociation. However, various studies have challenged these general characterizations of both WS (Karmiloff-Smith et al. 1997) and SLI (Johnston 1994; Leonard 1998) in terms of the clear distinction between spared and impaired aspects of functioning in language and cognitive domains. Further, the use of the neuropsychological model to investigate developmental disorders has been questioned on theoretical as well as empirical grounds (Bishop 1997, 1999; Juola and Plunkett 2000; Karmiloff-Smith 1997; Paterson et al. 1999). In an intriguing study reported in *Science,* Paterson and colleagues found that infants with WS performed relatively poorly on a language task but performed well on a task involving numerosity judgments. This is the reverse of the pattern seen in adults with WS, who have relatively good vocabulary abilities and poor number skills. These findings point to the danger in assuming that phenotypic outcomes involving uneven cognitive profiles observed in middle childhood or adulthood characterize infant starting states.

An alternate approach involves the use of experimental group design studies to explore particular aspects of functioning in children with varying language profiles. This is the approach that is frequently adopted by researchers whose main focus is to characterize the nature of developmental language disorders and who are secondarily concerned with utilizing atypical cases to inform theoretical models of normal cognitive processes. This is the tack that we have adopted in much of our research, which has examined cognitive and language abilities in specific language impairment. The term SLI (alternately, "specific language delay") has been used to refer to a group of children who demonstrate language disorders in the absence of any clearly identifiable etiology. Key features characterizing this population are delayed onset and acquisition of language, normal nonverbal intelligence, normal hearing, and absence of emotional disturbance (no evidence of pervasive developmental disorder, PDD) or frank neurological deficits. Normal range cognitive functioning has typically been defined as nonverbal IQ of 85 or higher, though there is renewed debate about the appropriate cut-off for normal cognitive range and about whether a language-cognitive discrepancy is critical to classification of SLI. This is a point that will be considered in more detail below.

Theoretical accounts of SLI can be divided into two general camps. Competence-based, linguistic accounts of the disorder have been proposed that postulate specific deficits within aspects of the grammatical system, such as the Extended Optional Infinitive account (Rice and Wexler 1996; Rice, Wexler, and Redmond 1999). This view stems from a nativist, generative grammar framework in which language is viewed as a modular facility; therefore, the focus is solely on the nature of grammatical deficits in SLI and characterization of cognitive abilities is not an issue. On the other hand, SLI has been viewed as a manifestation of a broader cognitive impairment within various Processing Limitation accounts. The nature and basis of these accounts varies from hypotheses about specific constraints in temporal processing or in phonological working memory to claims that linguistic deficits are secondary to more general information processing limitations. The impetus for appealing to a more broadly defined limited capacity framework is to attempt to capture the range of deficits exhibited by children with SLI. Despite the label "SLI," it is well documented that these children demonstrate certain cognitive limitations in addition to their deficits in linguistic skills, even though they perform within the normal range on standardized measures of nonverbal intelligence (cf. Leonard 1998). For example, children with SLI have been shown to perform significantly worse than matched controls on nonverbal tasks involving hypothesis testing, inference construction, and visual imagery or mental rotation. Within a general processing limitation framework, one could account for difficulties that children with SLI demonstrate in linguistic processing as well as limitations on certain nonverbal tasks by proposing that these children are restricted in their ability to simultaneously hold in mind and manipulate multiple pieces of information, especially when rapid processing is required.

There are a number of models of language processing that incorporate the notion of a limited capacity system; those proposed by Baddeley and colleagues (Baddeley 1986; 1998; Gathercole and

Baddeley 1993) and Just, Carpenter, and colleagues (Daneman and Carpenter 1980; Just and Carpenter 1992) have been most influential in language disorders research. Although the details of these theories vary, the central premise is that there is a limited pool of cognitive operational resources available to perform computations and when demands exceed available resources, processing and storage of linguistic information is degraded. Within this perspective, an individual's success in comprehending and producing language is dependent upon the ability to actively maintain and integrate linguistic material in working memory and trade-offs are thought to occur within and across language domains as demands reach the limits of available resources.

Support for limited capacity models of language processing comes from several sources. Evidence of linguistic interactions and trade-offs has been reported within the language acquisition literature. For instance, increased naming errors have been observed to co-occur with rapid growth in productive vocabulary and increased rates of speaking in young children (Gershkoff-Stowe and Smith 1997). Experimental studies with adults have also demonstrated trade-off effects, such that speed and accuracy of linguistic processing declines as cognitive load is increased. Factors that have been observed to affect linguistic processing include degree of lexical ambiguity, degree of syntactic complexity or ambiguity, and constraints in processing time (Carpenter and Just 1989; MacDonald, Just, and Carpenter 1992; Miyake, Carpenter, and Just 1994). A number of investigations have reported direct associations between working memory capacity and language abilities for children and adults. Specifically, research has revealed an association between phonological working memory and vocabulary development in young children (Baddeley, Gathercole, and Papagno 1998; Gathercole and Baddeley 1990, 1993). School-age children's performance on working memory measures has been found to be significantly correlated with spoken language comprehension and with reading recognition and comprehension (Ellis Weismer, Evans, and Hesketh 1999; Gaulin and Campbell 1994; Seigneuric et al. 2000; Swanson 1996). Working memory capacity has been shown to predict a number of verbal abilities in adults including reading comprehension levels, understanding of ambiguous passages and syntactically complex sentences and the ability to make inferences (Carpenter, Miayke, and Just 1994; Daneman and Carpenter 1980, 1983; King and Just 1991).

Evidence from children with language disorders, based on language sample data, indicates that they exhibit various types of linguistic trade-offs suggesting capacity constraints. For example, these children are more likely to make speech production errors and to omit words in longer, more grammatically complex sentences (Panagos and Prelock 1982). Children with SLI have also been found to make a disproportionate number of morphological errors compared to controls matched on mean length of utterance when producing utterances with high semantic complexity (Namazi and Johnston 1996). In prior experimental work, including some of our own research, limitations in processing capacity have been proposed to account for the poor performance of children with SLI in various areas, including deficient nonword repetition, poor novel word learning within sentences presented at fast speaking rates, and ineffective sentence comprehension processing (Edwards and Lahey 1998; Ellis Weismer and Hesketh 1996; Montgomery 1995, 2000). Building on this work, we sought to further examine the limited processing capacity account of SLI in these investigations.

The two studies summarized in this chapter were conducted as part of a longitudinal, epidemiologic investigation of SLI funded by the National Institutes of Health, directed by Dr. J. Bruce Tomblin, University of Iowa.[1] To establish this sample, a stratified cluster sampling procedure was used in which language abilities of 7,218 kindergarten children in rural, urban, and suburban areas of the upper Midwest were screened. Children who failed the screening (26%) and an equal number of controls were administered a diagnostic language battery using accepted diagnostic standards (Tomblin, Records, and Zhang 1996). Results indicated that the estimated prevalence rate for SLI in kindergarten is 7.4% (8% for boys and 6% for girls) (Tomblin et al. 1997). The 604 children who had been administered the full assessment protocol formed the sample who have been followed longitudinally by researchers from various universities as part of a project referred to as the Midwest Collaboration on Specific Language Impairment. For the studies described in this chapter, the data collection occurred when the children were in second and third grades.

In the first study (Ellis Weismer and Thordardottir 1999), we addressed two main questions. First, we asked whether performance on processing capacity measures accounts for significant variance in children's language abilities beyond that attributable to differences in nonverbal cognition. Secondly, we examined the role of nonverbal cognitive level in processing capacity limitations for children with language impairment. In this study we investigated performance of 134

[1]Funding for the studies reported in this chapter was provided by National Institutes of Deafness and Other Communicative Disorders (NIDCD), grant 5 P50 DC02746, "Midwest Collaboration on Specific Language Impairment" (J. Bruce Tomblin, Director; S. Ellis Weismer, Investigator). Preparation of this manuscript was partially supported by the continuation grant, "Collaboration on Specific Language Impairment."

children with varying levels of nonverbal cognitive abilities on three processing capacity measures; their scores ranged from 2 standard deviations below the mean to 2 standard deviations above the mean (i.e., nonverbal IQ scores of 70–130). Children from three language/ cognitive diagnostic categories were included in this study: (1) specific language impairment (SLI) group—normal range cognition (at least 85 IQ) but low language abilities; (2) nonspecific language impairment (NLI) group—low nonverbal cognition (70–84 IQ) and low language abilities; and (3) normal language (NL) controls—normal cognitive and language abilities.

As mentioned previously, the role of cognitive discrepancy criteria in defining SLI has recently come under scrutiny. Tager-Flusberg and Cooper (1999) have published a report based on an NIH-sponsored seminar on defining the phenotype of SLI. As they note in that report, dyslexia research has found the same basis for reading difficulty in children with a wide range of nonverbal IQs, leading to the elimination of nonverbal IQ level and discrepancy criteria in diagnosing reading impairment. Genetic research by Tomblin and Buckwalter (1998) has revealed similar heritability estimates for children with normal range nonverbal IQs and those with somewhat lower IQs. More recently, findings by Tomblin and Zhang (1999) for this same sample of children in the Iowa epidemiologic study have indicated that the basic language phenotype using standardized language measures is similar for children with language impairment whose nonverbal IQs fall above or below 85. These findings prompted us to examine the role of nonverbal cognitive level relative to processing capacity.

In these investigations we administered three processing capacity measures. We developed a Dual Processing Comprehension Task in which sentences (involving commands) are presented under competing and non-competing listening conditions. The children demonstrate their comprehension of the commands by manipulating the appropriate tokens. In the competing condition, primary and secondary sentences (distinguished by male/female speakers) are presented simultaneously. Children are instructed to respond first to the primary sentences (e.g., "Put the white square on the red circle") and then to the secondary sentences (e.g., "Touch the big boat and the little shoe"). These digitized sets of utterances are presented binaurally via headphones.

We also administered a version of a listening span measure, based on Daneman and Carpenter's (1980) listening span task, that was devised by Gaulin and Campbell (1994) to assess verbal working memory in typically developing children. This measure consists of sets of 1 to 6 short sentences. These simple sentences tap children's vocabulary and basic world knowledge. True/false responses are elicited following each sentence to ensure comprehension processing (e.g., "Sugar is sweet"—True, "Carrots can dance"—False). Concurrently, children are asked to recall the last word in each sentence (e.g., "sweet" and "dance") after all sentences in the set have been presented.

The third task was a nonword repetition task, assumed to be a measure of phonological processing capacity. This task was a version devised by Dollaghan (1995) and used by Dollaghan and Campbell (1998). The nonword repetition task consists of a set of 16 nonsense words ranging in length from 1syllable (e.g., "doif") to 4 syllables (e.g., "davonochig"), that children are asked to repeat immediately following the taped presentation of each item. The phonemes in the nonwords are early developing, acoustically salient sounds, stress patterns do not follow the typical English metrical stress pattern, and none of the syllables that make up the nonsense words correspond to actual English words.

It is important to note that although all of the processing capacity measures are restricted to linguistic processing and storage (verbal working memory), they do include controls for direct contributions of extant language knowledge. In the Dual Processing Comprehension Task, each child's competing condition performance was subtracted from the baseline level of sentence comprehension under non-competing listening conditions, resulting in a difference score. On the listening span measure, we analyzed word recall performance with and without the use of comprehension scores from the true/false items as a covariate (with the same results). The nonword repetition task consists of novel stimuli involving "low wordlikeness."

As shown in figure 1, hierarchical multiple regression analysis revealed that nonverbal cognitive scores combined with performance on processing measures predicted performance on a standardized measure of language comprehension and production ($r^2 = .41$, $p < .05$). The cognitive scores consisted of Performance IQs from the Wechsler Intelligence Scale for Children- III (Wechsler 1991) and language scores were based on the receptive and expressive subtests of the Clinical Evaluation of Language Fundamentals - 3 (Semel, Wiig, and Secord 1995). After the contribution of nonverbal cognition was accounted for (21% of the variance), each of the processing capacity measures added significant unique variance in language scores, though the listening span measure accounted for substantially more variance than the other two tasks. It is important to note the amount of variance left unaccounted for—clearly, processing capacity is not the entire story, a point we will return to later.

We then conducted group comparisons, excluding children who exhibited normal language skills at second grade but had a history of language delay. These comparisons revealed significant differences in

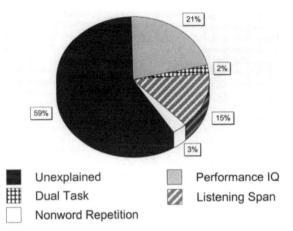

Figure 1. The amount of variance accounted for in children's performance on a standardized test of language comprehension and production, by performance IQ and the three processing capacity measures (Dual Processing Comprehension Task, Listening Span Task, Nonword Repetition Task).

processing capacity, as illustrated in figure 2. Children with SLI who met the cognitive discrepancy criterion (normal range nonverbal cognitive score of 85 or above, but low language abilities) performed significantly worse than controls on the Dual Processing Comprehension Task. The same pattern of results was found for analyses involving a broader definition of language impairment (LI) which included children with nonspecific language impairment who had low cognitive

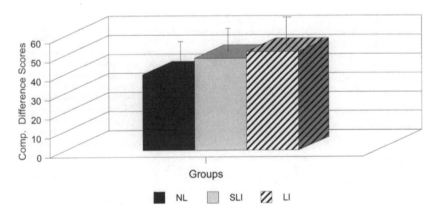

Figure 2. Mean comprehension difference scores on the Dual Processing Comprehension Task for the groups with normal language (NL), specific language impairment (SLI), and more broadly defined language impairment (LI).

abilities and low language skills and, therefore, did not meet the cognitive discrepancy criterion. As shown in figure 3, a similar pattern of results was found for the listening span task, in which both groups of children with language impairment were significantly worse than the NL controls but not significantly different from each other. Results for the nonword repetition task followed the same pattern, as illustrated in figure 4. Thus, the findings across these three processing capacity measures were highly consistent.

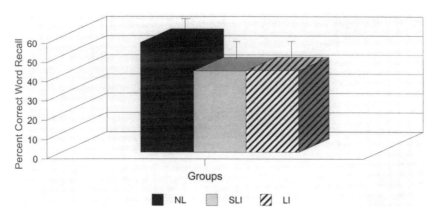

Figure 3.   Mean percent word recall on the Listening Span Task for the groups with normal language (NL), specific language impairment (SLI), and more broadly defined language impairment (LI).

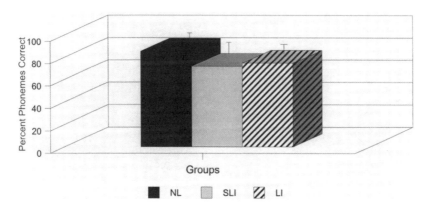

Figure 4.   Mean percent phonemes correct on the Nonword Repetition Task for the groups with normal language (NL), specific language impairment (SLI), and more broadly defined language impairment (LI).

The following conclusions can be drawn from this study. First, findings support claims of an association between processing capacity in verbal working memory and language abilities in school-age children. Secondly, although nonverbal IQ (along with processing capacity scores) was predictive of language ability for the group as a whole, nonverbal cognitive level did not distinguish between the children with language impairment in terms of processing capacity. Finally, children with language impairment, strictly defined or more broadly defined in terms of cognitive level, evidenced restrictions in linguistic processing capacity compared to age-matched peers with normal language.

In the second study (Ellis Weismer et al. 2000), we took a more in depth look at nonword repetition performance as an index of phonological processing capacity. There has been considerable interest in various versions of this measure in language and working memory studies with adults as well as with children. It has also gained widespread attention in the language disorders literature. Bishop and colleagues have suggested that nonword repetition provides a phenotypic marker of SLI based on genetic research utilizing twin methodology (Bishop, North, and Donlan 1996). Dollaghan and Campbell (1998) have also reported that their nonword repetition task may have clinical utility as a screening measure. Prior work has been based on smaller, clinically referred samples of children with language impairment. Given some of the findings from the area of dyslexia, we know that characterizations can differ between population-based samples and samples consisting of children who are selected based on clinical referral. Therefore, we sought to confirm our earlier findings from subsets of this sample regarding deficits in nonword repetition and to explore its clinical utility in ruling in and ruling out language problems in children from varying backgrounds.

The specific research questions addressed by this study were as follows: (1) Are there significant differences in nonword repetition for children grouped according to second grade diagnostic category, and if so, what is the nature of the differences? (2) How accurately do nonword repetition task scores rule in and rule out cases based on diagnostic category or treatment status? and (3) Is nonword repetition performance similar for children from different ethnic/cultural backgrounds? In this study we examined the nonword repetition performance of 581 children with and without language impairment (although all 604 children in the epidemiologic sample had been administered this task, 22 children whose performance IQs fell below 70 were excluded from this study along with one child whose audiotaped responses were unavailable due to technical difficulties). In addition to the groups we examined in the previous study, we also included a Low Cognition (LC) group. The LC group consisted of 53 children whose IQs were between 1 and 2 standard deviations below the mean, but who had normal range language abilities.

Results revealed significant group effects for total percentage phonemes correct, such that children with specific language impairment (SLI) and nonspecific language impairment (NLI) performed significantly worse than both normal language (NL) controls and the low cognition (LC) group (see figure 5). There was no statistically significant difference between the SLI and NLI groups or between the NL and LC groups. We then looked at the impact of stimulus complexity on performance; these findings are depicted in figure 6. Repeated

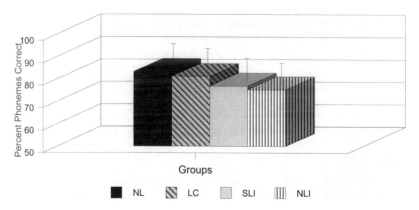

Figure 5. Diagnosis main effects: Mean percent phonemes correct on the Nonword Repetition Task for the diagnostic categories of normal language (NL), low cognition (LC), specific language impairment (SLI), and nonspecific language impairment (NLI).

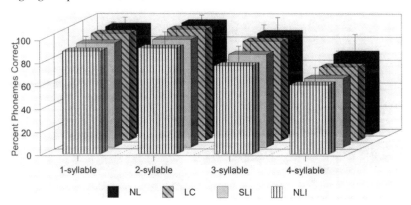

Figure 6. Diagnosis by syllable length effects: Mean percent phonemes correct on 1-, 2-, 3-, and 4-syllable targets on the Nonword Repetition Task for the diagnostic categories of normal language (NL), low cognition (LC), specific language impairment (SLI), and nonspecific language impairment (NLI).

measures analyses indicated a significant group (diagnosis) x syllable length interaction. Although the children with language impairment (SLI and NLI) performed worse than those with normal language at each syllable length, the largest group differences occurred on the 3- and 4-syllable nonwords. This increased difficulty with more complex targets exhibited by the children with language impairment is consistent with a processing capacity limitation interpretation. Although the low cognitive (LC) group outperformed children with language impairment at each syllable length, this difference did not reach statistical significance for 4-syllable nonwords.

To address the issue of whether nonword repetition performance has clinical utility in distinguishing between children with language disorder and those without, we employed Likelihood (LH) ratio analysis procedures (cf. Sackett et al. 1991), using second grade diagnosis or treatment status as the gold standard. Results indicated that children with SLI were $4^1/_2$ times more likely to obtain low nonword repetition scores (below 60% accuracy) than NL controls, and those with NLI were 4 times more likely than controls to have scores in this range. In terms of ruling out the disorder, LH ratios of less than 1 indicated that high scores (above 91%) were more likely to come from controls. The LH ratio analyses for treatment status, using these same cut points, revealed that children in therapy were 10 times more likely to obtain low nonword repetition scores than those not in treatment and that none of the scores of 91% or better came from children in treatment. In a final analysis, we examined the distribution of scores broken down by race/ethnicity and found that, unlike many standardized language tests, there was no evidence of cultural bias in the pattern of responses on the nonword repetition task.

To summarize, these results from a large, population-based sample confirm that children with language impairment (whether defined narrowly or more broadly with respect to nonverbal cognition) exhibit deficits in nonword repetition, indicating restricted phonological processing capacity. The findings further support the contention that nonword repetition performance may provide a non-biased index to assist in ruling in or ruling out language disorder in children from varying cultural backgrounds.

In conclusion, findings from this project indicate that children with language impairment evidenced significantly poorer performance on each of the processing capacity measures than typically developing controls with normal language skills. This was the case for children with specific language impairment (defined in terms of cognitive discrepancy criteria) as well as those with both low cognitive and low language skills. Further, the findings suggest that processing capacity measures may have clinical utility in distinguishing between children with and without language disorder. Overall, these results support the claim that capacity limitations in cognitive processing resources play a role in language disorders, though we do not view this research as attempting to identify THE cause of SLI. Like many researchers, we would ascribe to a model in which causal factors in language disorders are assumed be to heterogeneous, multifaceted, and interactive. That is, there are likely multiple, highly interactive factors at work that may operate differently for different children. Nevertheless, processing capacity limitations do appear to be a piece of the problem.

In future investigations we intend to explore the issue of the distinction between linguistic processing and verbal working memory in light of new theoretical frameworks that have been proposed (Mac-Donald and Christiansen 2002). We are also planning to examine whether children with SLI exhibit domain-specific or general processing capacity limitations, impacting processing of nonverbal as well as verbal stimuli. It should be noted that other investigators working on the Midwest Collaboration on SLI project with this same sample of children have found evidence that the children with language impairment exhibit reduced processing speed across modalities on a variety of tasks (Miller et al. 2001). In our future studies we will be comparing performance on a spatial working memory task to various linguistic processing and verbal working memory measures. Finally, we are currently using neuroimaging techniques (fMRI) with a small subset of the epidemiologic sample to assess whether children with language impairment exhibit atypical, reduced activation patterns on a linguistic processing and verbal working memory task.

The issues discussed in this chapter, related to IQ cutoff scores/ cognitive discrepancy criteria and the consideration of processing capacity limitations, have potential clinical implications for assessment and treatment of children with language impairment. There appears to be mounting evidence that cognitive discrepancy criteria may not be particularly useful in establishing a meaningful phenotype of developmental language disorder. Further, several studies have demonstrated that children with flat cognitive-language profiles benefit as much from language intervention as those with discrepant profiles, i.e., both display similar responsiveness to treatment (Cole, Coggins, and Vanderstoep 1999; Cole, Dale, and Mills 1990; Fey, Long, and Cleave 1994). If we suspect that processing capacity limitations underlie language impairment, then measures tapping processing abilities should be included in our diagnostic batteries. Processing measures provide an index of implementation of language skills in real-time communicative contexts that can at least be a useful adjunct to information gained from traditional, knowledge-based tests. Several studies have indicated that processing measures may be more useful than our standardized tests in distinguishing between language differences and disorders in children from culturally and linguistically diverse backgrounds (Campbell et al. 1997; Dollaghan and Campbell 1998). Treatment implications of limited processing capacity claims include paying attention to the manner in which linguistic models are presented, as well as the content, decreasing cognitive load by introducing new forms in highly familiar routines or scripts, and working to increase automaticity of newly acquired language skills before advancing to new goals (cf. Ellis Weismer 1996, 2000). Consideration of processing limitations may also be useful in early identification of children at risk for language impairment and in prediction of language outcomes. We are exploring this possibility in an ongoing longitudinal investigation[2] of the link between late onset of language development in toddlers and SLI (Ellis Weismer and Evans 2002). Advancing our understanding of the nature of the relationship between language and cognition in children with language disorder is not only of interest from a theoretical perspective, but may have important implications for diagnosis, prognosis, and treatment of children with language deficits.

REFERENCES

Baddeley, A. 1986. *Working Memory.* Oxford, England: Claredon Press.

Baddeley, A. 1998. *Human Memory: Theory and Practice* (rev. ed.). Boston: Allyn & Bacon.

Baddeley, A., Gathercole, S., and Papagno, C. 1998. The phonological loop as a language learning device. *Psychological Review* 105:158–73.

Bishop, D.V.M. 1997. Cognitive neuropsychology and developmental disorders: Uncomfortable bedfellows. *Quarterly Journal of Experimental Psychology* 50A: 899–923

Bishop, D.V.M. 1999. An innate basis for language? *Science* 286:2283–4.

Bishop, D.V.M., North, T., and Donlan, C. 1996. Nonword repetition as a behavioural marker for inherited language impairment: Evidence from a twin study. *Journal of Child Psychology and Psychiatry* 37:391–403.

Campbell, T., Dollaghan, C., Needleman, H., and Janosky, J. 1997. Reducing bias in language assessment: Processing-dependent measures. *Journal of Speech, Language, and Hearing Research* 40:519–25.

[2]Support for the longitudinal investigation of the link between late onset of language in toddlers and specific language impairment is being provided by NIDCD grant 5 R01 DC03731, "Linguistic Processing in Specific Language Delay" (S. Ellis Weismer, Principal Investigator; J. Evans and R. Chapman, Co-PIs). Partial support for the preparation of this manuscript also came from this grant.

Carpenter, P., and Just, M. 1989. The role of working memory in language comprehension. In *Complex Information Processing: The Impact of Herbert A. Simon*, eds. D. Klahr and K. Kotovsky. Hillsdale, NJ: Lawrence Erlbaum Associates.

Carpenter, P., Miyake, A., and Just, M. 1994. Working memory constraints in comprehension: Evidence from individual differences, aphasia, and aging. In *Handbook of Psycholinguistics*, ed. M.A. Gernsbacher. San Diego: Academic Press.

Chomsky, N. 1964. Current issues in linguistic theory. In *The Structure of Language: A Philosophical Approach to Language Based on Selected Articles Dealing with the Theories, Methods, and Results of Linguistics*, eds. J. A. Fodor and J. J. Katts. Englewoods, NJ: Prentice Hall.

Chomsky, N. 1988. *Language and Problems of Knowledge: The Managua Lectures*. Cambridge, MA: MIT Press.

Cole, K., Coggins, T., and Vanderstoep, C. 1999. The influence of language/cognitive profile on discourse intervention outcome. *Language, Speech and Hearing Services in Schools* 30:61–67.

Cole, K., Dale, P., and Mills, P. 1990. Defining language delay in young children by cognitive referencing: Are we saying more than we know? *Applied Psycholinguistics* 11:292–302.

Daneman, M., and Carpenter, P. 1980. Individual differences in working memory and reading. *Journal of Verbal Learning and Verbal Behavior* 19:450–66.

Daneman, M., and Carpenter, P. 1983. Individual differences in integrating information between and within sentences. *Journal of Experimental Psychology: Learning, Memory and Cognition* 9:561–83.

Dollaghan, C. 1995. Nonword Reptition Task (NRT). Unpublished assessment measure.

Dollaghan, C., and Campbell, T. 1998. Nonword repetition and child language impairment. *Journal of Speech, Language, and Hearing Research* 41:1136–46.

Edwards, J., and Lahey, M. 1998. Nonword repetitions of children with specific language impairment: Exploration of some explanations for their inaccuracies. *Applied Psycholinguistics* 19:279–309.

Ellis Weismer, S. 1996. Capacity limitations in working memory: The impact on lexical and morphological learning by children with language impairment. *Topics in Language Disorders* 17:33–44.

Ellis Weismer, S. 2000. Intervention for children with developmental language delay. In *Speech and Language Impairments*, eds. D.V. M. Bishop and L. Leonard. Hove, East Sussex: Psychology Press.

Ellis Weismer, S., and Elin T. Thordardottir. 1999. Verbal working memory abilities of school-age children with and without language impairment. Poster presented at the biennial meeting of the Society for Research in Child Development, Albuquerque, New Mexico, April.

Ellis Weismer, S., and Evans, J. 2002. The role of processing limitations in early identification of specific language impairment. *Topics in Language Disorders* 22:15–29.

Ellis Weismer, S., Evans, J., and Hesketh, L. 1999. Examination of verbal working memory capacity in children with specific language impairment. *Journal of Speech, Language, and Hearing Research* 42:1249–60.

Ellis Weismer, S., and Heskcth, L. 1996. Lexical learning by children with specific language impairment: Effects of linguistic input presented at varying speaking rates. *Journal of Speech, Language, and Hearing Research* 39:177–90.

Ellis Weismer, S., Tomblin, J. B., Zhang, X., Buckwalter, P., Chynoweth, J. G., and Jones, M. 2000. Nonword repetition performance in school-age children with and without language impairment. *Journal of Speech, Language, and Hearing Research* 43:865–78.

Fey, M., Long, S., and Cleave, P. 1994. Reconsideration of IQ criteria in the definition of specific language impairment. In *Communication and Language Intervention Series, Vol. 4: Specific Language Impairments in Children*, eds. R. Watkins and M. Rice. Baltimore: Brookes.

Fodor, J. A. 1983. *The Modularity of Mind.* Cambridge, MA: Bradford Books.

Gathercole, S., and Baddeley, A. 1990. The role of phonological memory in vocabulary acquisition: A study of young children learning new words. *British Journal of Psychology* 81:439–54.

Gathercole, S., and Baddeley, A. 1993. *Working Memory and Language Processing.* Hillsdale, NJ: Lawrence Erlbaum Associates.

Gaulin, C., and Campbell, T. 1994. Procedure for assessing verbal working memory in normal school-age children: Some preliminary data. *Perceptual and Motor Skills* 79:55–64.

Gershkoff-Stowe, L., and Smith, L. B. 1997. A curvilinear trend in naming errors as a function of early vocabulary growth. *Cognitive Psychology* 34:37–71.

Johnston, J. 1994. Cognitive abilities of children with language impairment. In *Communication and Language Intervention Series, Vol. 4: Specific Language Impairments in Children*, eds. R. Watkins and M. Rice. Baltimore: Brookes.

Juola, P., and Plunkett, K. 2000. Why double dissociations don't mean much. In *Exploring Cognition: Damaged Brains and Neural Networks: Readings in Cognitive Neuropsychology and Connectionist Modeling*, eds. G. Cohen and R.A. Johnston. Philadelphia: Psychology Press.

Just, M., and Carpenter, P. 1992. A capacity theory of comprehension: Individual differences in working memory. *Psychological Review* 99:122–49.

Karmiloff-smith, A., Grant, J., Berthoud, I., Davies, M., Howlin, P., and Udwin, O. 1997. Language and Williams syndrome: How intact is "intact"? *Child Development* 68:246–62.

King, J., and Just, M. 1991. Individual differences in syntactic processing: The role of working memory. *Journal of Memory and Language* 30:580–602.

Leonard, L. 1998. *Children with Specific Language Impairment.* Cambridge, MA: MIT Press.

MacDonald, M. C., Just, M., and Carpenter, P. 1992. Working memory constraints on the processing of syntactic ambiguity. *Cognitive Psychology* 24:56–98.

MacDonald, M. C., and Christiansen, M. H. 2002. Reassessing working memory: Comment on Just & Carpenter (1992) and Waters & Caplan (1996). *Psychological Review* 109:35–54.

MacWhinney, B., ed. 1999. *The Emergence of Language.* Mahwah, NJ: Lawrence Erlbaum Associates.

Miller, C. A., Kail, R., Leonard, L., and Tomblin, J. B. 2001. Speed of processing in children with specific language impairment. *Journal of Speech, Language, and Hearing Research* 44: 416–33.

Miyake, A., Carpenter, P., and Just, M. 1994. A capacity approach to syntactic comprehension disorders: Making normal adults perform like aphasic patients. *Cognitive Neuropsychology* 11:671–717.

Montgomery, J. 1995. Sentence comprehension in children with specific language impairment: The role of phonological working memory. *Journal of Speech and Hearing Research* 38:177–89.

Montgomery, J. 2000. Verbal working memory and sentence comprehension in children with specific language impairment. *Journal of Speech, Language and Hearing Research* 43:293–308.

Namazi, M., and Johnston, J. 1996. The relationship between grammatical morphology and semantic complexity in the utterances of language-impaired children. Poster presented at the Symposium on Research in Child Language Disorders, Madison, Wisconsin, June.

Panagos, J., and Prelock, P. 1982. Phonological constraints on the sentence productions of language-disordered children. *Journal of Speech and Hearing Research* 25:171–77.

Paterson, S., Brown, J., Gsîdl, M., Johnson, M., and Karmiloff-Smith, A. 1999. Cognitive modularity and genetic disorders. *Science* 286: 2355–8.

Pinker, S. 1994. *The Language Instinct.* New York: William Morrow and Company, Inc.

Rice, M., and Wexler, K. 1996. Toward tense as a clinical marker of specific language impairment in English-speaking children. *Journal of Speech and Hearing Research* 39:1239–57.

Rice, M., Wexler, K., and Redmond, S. 1999. Grammaticality judgments of an extended optional infinitive grammar: Evidence from English-speaking children with specific language impairment. *Journal of Speech, Language, and Hearing Research* 42:943–61.

Sackett, D., Haynes, R., Guyatt, G., and Tugwell, P. 1991. *Clinical Epidemiology: A Basic Science for Clinical Medicine.* Boston: Little, Brown.

Seigneuric, A., Ehrlich, M. F., Oakhill, J., and Yuill, N. 2000. Working memory resources and children's reading comprehension. *Reading and Writing* 13:81–103.

Semel, E., Wiig, E., and Secord, W. 1995. *Clinical Evaluation of Language Fundamentals-3 (CELF-3).* San Antonio, TX: Psychological Corporation.

Swanson, H. L. 1996. Individual and age-related differences in children's working memory. *Memory and Cognition* 24:70–82.

Tager-Flusberg, H., and Cooper, J. 1999. Present and future possibilities for defining a phenotype for specific language impairment. *Journal of Speech, Language, and Hearing Research* 42:1275–8.

Tomblin, J. B., and Buckwalter, P. 1998. Heritability of poor language achievement among twins. *Journal of Speech, Language, and Hearing Research* 41:188–99.

Tomblin, J. B., Records, N., Buckwalter, P., Zhang, X., Smith, E., and O'Brien, M. 1997. Prevalence of specific language impairment in kindergarten children. *Journal of Speech, Language, and Hearing Research* 40:1245–60.

Tomblin, J. B., Records, N., and Zhang, X. 1996. A system for the diagnosis of specific language impairment in kindergarten. *Journal of Speech and Hearing Research* 39:1284–94.

Tomblin, J. B., and Zhang, X. 1999. Language patterns and etiology in children with specific language impairment. In *Neurodevelopmental Disorders: Developmental Cognitive Neuroscience,* ed. H. Tager-Flusberg. Cambridge, MA: MIT Press.

Wechsler, D. 1991. *Wechsler Intelligence Scale for Children-III (WISC-III).* San Antonio, TX: Psychological Corporation.

Chapter • 3

Language Development: Does the Environment Matter?

Betty Hart

The environment of language development is the social dance created when people talk together. Talking using words or signs is the social purpose of learning language. From listening to their children talk, parents learn whether their children are making progress—or are failing to do so.

Beginning to talk, like starting to walk, is so predictably a part of human development that we are challenged to account for instances when children have problems (Menyuk 1975). As Locke notes,

> We know something about WHEN the typical infant begins to talk. And we know WHICH infants are late to begin. It would be nice if clinicians could help slowly developing children catch up with their peers, but we do not know—do not even have a clue, if the truth be known—as to WHY the typical infant begins to talk, much less why most of the late ones are several steps behind (1996, p.252; caps in the original).

Addressing the WHY question requires longitudinal data (Miller 1987) that enable comparing the beginnings of talking across children. Just such data were available from two methodologically identical longitudinal studies that recorded the everyday social interactions of typically developing children learning to talk and comparison data from children with Down syndrome who were significantly delayed.

LONGITUDINAL DATA

In the first study (Hart and Risley 1995), typically developing children were observed from an average age of 9-months old until 3-years old in 42 families varied in size, race, and socioeconomic status. In the second study (Hart 1996), children with Down syndrome were observed from age 1 year until age 5 years in 11 families. The methods and data analysis were identical in the two studies (see Hart and Risley 1995 for details). For an hour each month, an observer carrying a tape recorder followed a child while making continuous notes concerning what the child was doing, with what, where, and with whom. The observer's notes and the tape recorded utterances were meshed during transcription, and the transcripts submitted to a series of computer programs for coding and analysis.

When families were recruited for the two studies, they were specifically asked to do just what they usually did when at home with the child. Because virtually all children learn to talk, whether their parents are illiterate or have advanced degrees, parents must be doing something that effectively supports language development even when they are not trying. The aim of the longitudinal studies was to find out what parents do in the course of everyday caregiving that encourages children to talk.

For several years, then, the observers recorded episodes of routine care—dressing, eating, toileting—plus frequent occasions of parents managing children while making the beds and folding the laundry, interspersed with bouts of joint activity: looking at a book, playing a game, picking up toys, or just gazing out the window. We saw, as we expected, the mutual responsiveness of frequent turn-taking (Bruner 1983; Bullowa 1979). Unexpected was finding that the great majority of what the children said, and their parents answered for months after the children began to say occasional words, were nonword utterances (vocalizations, babble, jargon, gibberish, intonational sentences).

We wondered at the role of nonword utterances during turn-taking, especially when we saw the high rates recorded among the children with Down syndrome. We wondered what a typical rate of vocalizations was and whether there might be an association with "why it is so hard for the child to learn words during the prelinguistic period" (Gelman 1983, p. 277).

THE TYPICAL PATTERN OF LEARNING TO TALK

We had averaged the data of the 42 typically developing children in order to examine the typical pattern of learning to talk (see figure 1) which we then described in terms of three phases (Hart and Risley 1999).

The Prelinguistic Period

The prelinguistic phase began at the children's first words at an average age of 11 months old. Marking the end of the phase was, along with a 50-word recorded vocabulary on average, a word spurt after the month that a child first produced as many or more word utterances as nonword utterances in an hour, an average of about 100 of each. An average delay before producing as many word utterances as nonwords utterances in an hour was 8 months, but a delay as long as 14 months—more than a year—was seen for 3 of the typically developing children, and more than 2 years for 2 of the children with Down syndrome.

The data illustrated Snow's (1988) observation that,

> It is striking how fragile are the first 10 to 15 words, and with what difficulty they are acquired. Only after a lexicon of 40 to 50 words is attained do children really become efficient word learners. Before that, each word represents a long and difficult process (p. 348).

Our observations showed us some aspects of parent-child interactions that seemed to be contributing to children's difficulties.

Making for difficulty. One factor that seemed to contribute to a delay in attaining a 40 to 50 word vocabulary was that although the children could have said, "Uhoh" or "Hi" 100 times an hour instead of vocalizing or speaking in gibberish, none of them did. Word and social context were apparently learned together (Harris et al. 1988), so that children said "Hi" only in a context of greeting, and "Bottle" was always a referent—or at least the parents always interpreted it as such.

The absence of any need or demand for words was also seen as contributing to a delay in producing as many word as nonword utterances during interactions. Parents said, "Say juice," and gave the children a cup at the same time. All the children's wants and needs, physical and social, were satisfied, whether the children vocalized, said a word, or were silent.

Further, the parents continued to do what they had been doing for a year. They often and actively encouraged the children to take a turn using nonwords, creating the conversations described by Snow (1977, p.20) in which parents "treat any response on the part of the child as a communicative response." Even though parents were more likely to answer when the children said words, they continued to respond regularly, and to engage in extended bouts of turn-taking, when 95% of the children's responses were gibberish.

Further contributing to a delay was the environment of interaction. For a 1-year-old who does not need words, answering with a word during interaction presents a formidable task (see Dapretto and Bjork 2000).

The child has to process an incoming utterance: *What* means a name is wanted. *That* means the name wanted is the name of the object the parent is looking at. The child has to check the parent's gaze, and then search the current lexicon for a corresponding entry, retrieve the phonemes, put them in the right linear order, and articulate them. And get all this done within the second or so before the parent decides the child does not know, and says, "That's a dog." For the child, how much easier just to say a nonword, "Ehnan," so that the parent can go ahead and take another turn.

While the parents waited for working memory, articulation, and vocabulary to grow, they had little alternative to maintaining, even sometimes encouraging, behaviors, babble, and gibberish, which would be socially unproductive in the long term.

The parents had to keep the children responding or they would lose social interaction. They would lose the immediate purpose for developing language. At first they gladly responded to repetitions and encouraged imitation, so that the children would find words as easy to produce as nonwords in the second or two the children had to take a turn. The parents needed the children to use enough words so that the parents could begin responding preferentially to variety, without risking that the children would drop back to using the vocalizations that continued to function effectively for maintaining interaction.

A Developmental Milestone. The phase change we saw in the data came when half or more of what the children said during interactions contained recognizable words. The children were an average of 19 months old, an age at which a word spurt is seen for many children. Not all children show a word spurt (Goldfield and Reznick 1990), but when a word spurt is seen it is interpreted as indicating the onset of multi-word utterances preceding syntax (Dromi 1987) and as the transition from prelinguistic to linguistic behavior (Gelman 1983). Because a word spurt marks a developmental milestone, it represents important evidence that the environment of interaction has changed in such a way that words predominate in children's responses.

The longitudinal data showed that the parents were responding, however, not just to the increasing frequency that their children answered using words during interactions, but to a combination of indices. The words the children were using displayed a variety of vocabulary indicative of cognitive development. The fluency of their answers indicated advances in memory and articulation. Progress in language development was indicated by the children's use of filler

syllables (see Veneziano and Sinclair 2000), combining bits of gibberish with words in order to reproduce the prosody of the language so
as to sound as if they were speaking English before they had the
words to make multi-word utterances.

The children's display of increasing ability and interest in speaking English led to an environment of frequent social dancing which
we characterized as Staying and Playing.

Staying and Playing

For the next 8 months on average, the parents and children were observed just staying with one another, the parents rediscovering the
wonder of the world through their children's words, and the children
blossoming in their parents' enjoyment. All the parent behaviors
shown in many, many studies to facilitate language development appeared in the parents' talk: expansions, extensions, and recasts of the
children's utterances, semantic matching, topic maintenance (Nelson
1973; Snow 1986). In figure 1 may be seen the acceleration in child
word utterances during these 8 months. The children's increasing fluency and elaboration naturally called for increasingly complex responses from their parents. The curriculum advanced automatically
with the sophistication of the social dance.

Matching the Family

Then, when the children were an average of 28 months old, they
began talking as much as other family members. Their parents
abruptly took on the role of listeners and the children's rates of talking
leveled off at the amount usual in the family, an amount similar to the
amount of parent talk addressed to the children during the first 8-
month phase (see figure 1). The children no longer needed encourage-
ment to talk. An occasional "Uhhuh" from the parent was enough to
keep the children describing in detail what the parents had just seen
them do, what the parents were currently watching them do, and
what the parents could safely predict that the children would do next.

Finding that the amount the children talked stopped accelerating
when the amount matched the amount usual in the family was as unexpected as was finding how vastly different ordinary American families are in how much talking goes on during the day. The average
number of utterances addressed to the children per hour was 341. The
range was from a parent who addressed an average of 54 utterances
per hour to the child to a parent who, on average, every month for
$2^{1}/_2$ years, addressed more than 800 utterances an hour to the child.

The children in the more taciturn families presumably could
have talked as much as the most talkative of the children, but they

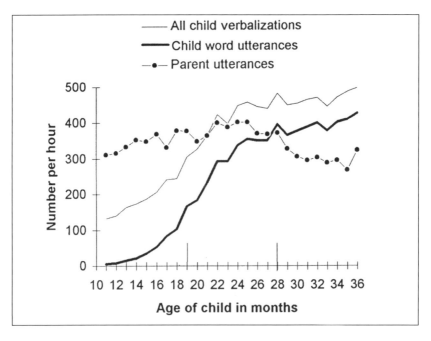

Figure 1. Average number per hour of parent (line with circles) and child verbalizations during the months the children were 11–36 months old. The light line shows all child verbalizations (word utterances plus nonword utterances) and the heavy line shows child word utterances (utterances containing recognizable words).

didn't. Their rates of talking leveled off at amounts similar to the family rate (see Hart and Risley 1999).

MEANINGFUL DIFFERENCES

The longitudinal data revealed major differences in the amount of children's language experience (Hart and Risley 1995). Clear in figure 2 is that the children were not only benefiting from their parents talking to them, they were actively contributing to their own language experience (see also Bloom 1991). Because experience is cumulative, the differences between the children were increasing with every month of family interaction.

Analysis revealed a highly significant correlation between parent talkativeness and child language outcomes measured at age 3 and at age 9 to 10. Parent talkativeness—an amount matched by the child—accounted for all the correlation between socioeconomic status and/or race and the children's accomplishments at age 3 in terms of vocabulary

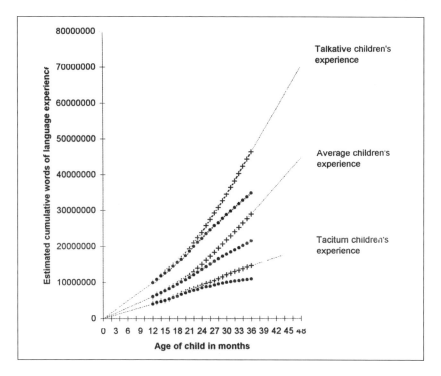

Figure 2. Estimated cumulative number of words of children's total language experience, assuming 14 hours per day or 100 hours per week of experience time. Exposure from the parent (lines with circles) is the cumulative number per hour of words said to each child by their parents. Added to exposure from the parent is the children's practice (lines with plus signs), the cumulative number per hour of words said by each child during each monthly in-home observation when the children were 12–36 months old. The dotted line trajectories were extrapolated back to birth from the parent exposure slopes and forward to 48 months of child age from the combined parent exposure and child practice slopes, to display an estimate of the increasing differences between talkative and taciturn families in the cumulative total language experience of their children. For description of the 4 talkative and the 4 taciturn children see Hart and Risley 1995.

growth rate, different words used per hour, score on the Stanford-Binet IQ test (Terman and Merrill 1960) and, at age 9 to10, in terms of scores on the Peabody Picture Vocabulary Test (Dunn and Dunn 1981) and the Test of Oral Language Development (Hammill and Newcomer 1988).

A strong relationship between parent talkativeness and child vocabulary growth results when parents talk spontaneously with their children as they go about their everyday activities. The continually changing context within and across those activities ensures continual variety in what is talked about. Parents casually mention to their children what is worth noticing about experience and what is worth naming and remembering. Parents do not need to monitor what they say or invest in a college education in order to provide their children with all the basic vocabulary that later words and concepts will build on and elaborate. For children whose vocabularies are starting from zero, all language, plain and fancy, is useful.

And the more parents talk with their children, the more often such facilitating behaviors as semantic matching and recasts occur to encourage the children to talk, and thus inform their parents about the children's progress in developing language, so that the curriculum can advance. Once talking gets started and parents and children begin to share in the social dances of conversation, what matters most is the amount of dancing that goes on. Exposure and practice come together in a partnership that facilitates language development.

The natural environment that supports learning to talk is the social dance that all parents do effectively when they are not doing anything deliberately. But if children who do not need words find words difficult to learn and hard to produce, getting the dance started may take a long time.

DELAY

In the longitudinal data of the children with Down syndrome, the pattern of learning to talk was similar to that seen in the data of the typically developing children. A prelinguistic period was followed by a period of staying and playing during which the children's rates of talking increased to match and then level off at the amount of talking customary in the family. Different across the children and data sets was the duration of the prelinguistic period. The longer the delay in attaining the milestone of producing as many word as nonword utterances during interaction, the more postponed was the period of staying and playing with its contexts for rapid and efficient word learning.

As Cicchetti and Beeghly note, "the study of Down syndrome can inform us about which stages, sequences, and structures are logically necessary . . . to the developmental process" (1990, p. 33). The longitudinal data offered a unique opportunity to inquire into Locke's (1996) question as to why infants begin to use words instead of continuing to communicate effectively using nonwords. We could look at what was happening in children's lives that was (or was not) associated with a lengthening delay in attaining the milestone of producing as many word as nonword utterances during interaction. We could compare data from the average among the typically developing children to both the data of the late talkers among the typically developing children and the data of the children with Down syndrome.

Data Compared

Average among the typically developing children were the 24 (12 boys, 12 girls) for whom the prelinguistic period lasted 8 months from the children's first words at an average age of 11 months until they attained the milestone of producing as many word as nonword utterances during interactions when they were an average age of 17 months. At the month before the milestone month, the average vocabulary recorded for the 24 children listed 50 words. Of their utterances during interactions that month, 27% combined words with nonword filler syllables.

The late talkers among the typically developing children were the 7 (4 girls, 3 boys) for whom the prelinguistic period lasted longest, an average of 12 months from the children's first words at an average age of 10 months until they attained the milestone of producing as many word as nonword utterances during interaction when they were an average age of 22 months. At the month before the milestone month the average vocabulary recorded for the 7 children listed 86 words. Of their utterances during interactions that month, 34% combined words with nonword filler syllables.

These 7 children seemed to represent the upper end of the normal curve. All their parents were told by their pediatricians not to worry that the children were not talking yet, and, like other late talkers (Thal, Tobias, and Morrison 1991), once the 7 children attained the milestone, they soon caught up to the average.

Anecdotally, the 7 children seemed to be cases of the kind of mismatch described by Nelson (1973), a high-rate parent perhaps overstimulating a low-rate child, or a high-rate child perhaps harrying a low-rate parent. It took time for them to work out how much dancing was acceptable to them both. They showed us, though, how much give there is in the natural environment that supports learning to talk, the range of variation in early experience that can be accommodated without prejudicing development.

The children with Down syndrome were the 5 (3 boys, 2 girls) for whom the prelinguistic period lasted 17–30 months, 22 months on average, from the month of the children's first words at an average age of 16 months until they attained the milestone of producing as many word utterances as nonword utterances during interactions when they were an average age of 41 months. At the month before the milestone month, the average vocabulary recorded for the 5 children listed 110 words. Of their utterances during interactions that month, 26% combined words with nonword filler syllables.

Set aside in this exploratory analysis were the data of the children for whom the prelinguistic period differed in length from the averages of the three groups under study. Then because of the differences in the numbers of months the children in the three groups spent in the prelinguistic period, averages were obtained for each of the three groups for the first three data months (for each child, the month of recording the first word and the next two months) and the last three data months (for each child, the month before the milestone month of recording as many word as nonword utterances during interactions, and the two prior months).

Similarities across the groups. The children's language development, the parents' behavior, and the environment of interaction were similar across the three groups.

As many other studies have shown (see Fowler 1990), the language development of the 5 children with Down syndrome was following a typical course. The 5 children with Down syndrome, like the late talkers, continued to learn new vocabulary such that the more the average months in the prelinguistic period, the larger the average recorded vocabulary. The developmental progress indicated by the children's increasing use of filler syllables was similar across the three groups. Like the typically developing children, the 5 children with Down syndrome were matching the prosody of the language, blending the hard words with the easy nonwords in order to sound as though they were speaking English.

All the parents were differentially responsive to word utterances (see figure 3). In the first three months of the prelinguistic period, the parents responded to an average of 89% to 92% of the word utterances the children produced during interactions and to an average of 61% to 74% of the nonword utterances the children produced during interactions. In the last three months of the prelinguistic period, the parents responded to an average of 83% to 90% of the word utterances the children produced during interactions and to an average of 68% to 80% of the nonword utterances the children produced.

Parents' greater responsiveness to word utterances than to nonword utterances was similar both across the three groups and over time, and did not change either as the prelinguistic period lengthened or as child responses increased (see figure 3).

Also similar across the three groups during the last three months of the prelinguistic period was the frequency of initiations. As though connected to some sort of biological clock, the parents and children in all three groups contacted one another on average about once per minute, 53 to 63 times an hour. Also, in all three groups, roughly half of such contacts seemed to be "just checking." Of all the initiations of contact, only about half, an average of 47% to 56%, led to episodes of interaction in which a child answered a parent utterance and got an answer from the parent.

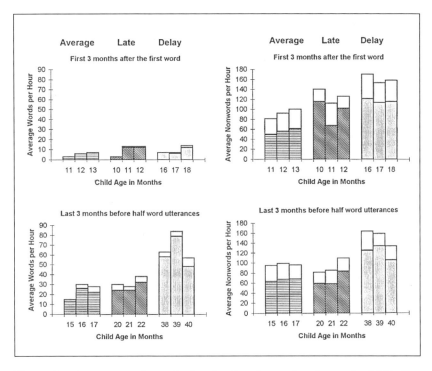

Figure 3.   Average per hour during the first 3 months after each child's first word (top panels) and during the last 3 months before half of the child's utterances during interactions contained recognizable words (bottom panels) of child word utterances (left panels) and nonword utterances (right panels) that the parent responded to (filled portions of bars) and did not respond to (open portions of bars). The three groups of children are: Average typically developing children (leftmost striped bars, n = 24), Late talker typically developing children (middle medium shaded bars, n = 7), and Delayed children with Down syndrome (rightmost light shaded bars, n = 5). Note the differing average ages in the 3 groups.

Of this subset of interactions (those involving mutual responses; see figure 3) slightly over half, 56%, were initiated by the parents in the two groups of typically developing children. The parents of the 5 children with Down syndrome initiated somewhat fewer, 45%, of interactions. In all three groups, three quarters of the interactions, 64% to 71%, ended when the children did not respond within 5 seconds. The parents could nearly always find something to say, even in response to a nonword utterance, in order to keep interaction going.

Also similar across the groups was parent help to get the dance started. The parents encouraged strategies that made words as easy to produce as nonwords. They modeled the ease and acceptability of repetition and imitation. They presented learning materials especially designed to attract toddlers to basic words and concepts. They rehearsed the same words over and over (the names of animals and body parts) and they made nonwords work as words when they asked, "What does a cow - a sheep - a cat - say?"

They arranged the social environment to prompt words. They spent time in joint activities, looking at books or magazines with the children, sharing a SeeNSay, doing a puzzle. In all three groups, similar to the findings in many other studies (see Moerk 1989 for review), during joint activities higher percentages of the children's responses contained words, 5% to 7% more. Words were prompted by the activity, by the familiarity of the materials and the words that named them, by the parents' enjoyment, as well as by the parents' words.

Across the three groups, the children's language development was similar, the parents' behaviors were similar, and the social environments of early childhood were similar.

Differences across the groups. The children's rates of using nonwords in the first three months of the prelinguistic period were strikingly different across the three groups (see figure 3). The higher the rate at which children produced nonword utterances during interaction, the more months it took to match that rate with word utterances. The 24 typically developing children at 17 months needed to answer 70 times or so using word utterances in order for half their responses during interactions to contain words. In contrast the 5 children with Down syndrome at 40 months needed to answer more than 100 times using word utterances, half again as often, so it is not surprising that they needed more months.

Among the 7 late talkers, the average rate of answering with nonword utterances during interactions decreased from an average of around 100 to an average around 80, similar to the rates of the 24 average children. The children's rates of responding, which in the first three months were more similar to the rates of the 5 children with Down syndrome, were in the last three months more similar to the rates of the 24 average children. Nonword utterances decreased because responding decreased, presumably as the parents and children were coming to agree on how much dancing they found comfortable. No such decline is seen in the data of the 5 children with Down syndrome during the three months before the milestone (see figure 3), nor was a systematic decline seen in the intervening months of data.

Interaction Context

When the 5 children with Down syndrome said their first words, their average rates of responding using nonwords during interactions were already twice the average rates of the 24 typically developing children (see figure 3). The higher rates may be seen to be a natural outcome of the longer and more frequent interactions needed for caring for the children with Down syndrome, and especially of the children's need for sensory and social stimulation (Roach et al. 1987). Their parents stimulated the children much more frequently, prompting and encouraging them to take a turn, treating a nonword utterance as an answer that enabled the parent to take another turn.

The children's need for stimulation did not change when the children began saying words. The children did not become more likely to get engaged independently or to maintain attention without parent guidance. Just as for the typically developing children, word utterances did not displace nonword utterances. Words were added like a second language, without reducing the rate of responding with a nonword utterance, or the usefulness of nonwords for getting a parent response.

Associated with the higher rates of responding for the 5 children with Down syndrome were more frequent and longer episodes of joint activity. When caregiving interactions during these last three months were excluded, when eating, dressing, and toileting were not topics, there remained about 45 to 50 minutes of an observation hour when the circumstances, the topics, and the length of interactions were optional. Of such optional interactions, the five children with Down syndrome spent an average of almost 60%, more than half, in joint activities, in contrast to the 20% average among the 24 typically developing children. The 5 children with Down syndrome were engaged in joint activity 3 times as often as the 24 typically developing children and they took twice as many turns. They averaged 10 responses per episode of joint activity. The average for the 24 typically developing children was 5.

For the 24 typically developing children, in contrast to the 5 children with Down syndrome, an average of 80% of the noncaregiving interactions during these last three months were concerned solely with taking care of the business of daily living, parents getting the children engaged, finding out what toy was wanted and delivering it, redirecting the children, managing transitions. Parents said, "Why don't you go get a toy?" "Are you wet?" "Go put that in the trash." In all three groups such interactions usually lasted only long enough to take care of the business at hand, an average of 2 to 3 child turns. Often few words were called for from the child. Increasingly often, the children merely responded, "No," regardless of what the parent said.

For the 24 typically developing children the continually changing locations and activities that became occasions for managing growing children led to continual variety in what was said. In the last three months before the milestone month, the 24 typically developing children, with an average recorded vocabulary approaching 50 words, used an average of 21 different words per hour. Almost half, 43%, were said in initiations or in response to someone other than the parent.

For the 5 children with Down syndrome, the more focused contexts of joint activity led to a more restricted range of topics, especially when similar learning materials were used over time. In the last three months before the milestone month the 5 children with Down syndrome, with an average recorded vocabulary approaching 110 words, used an average of 28 different words per hour, 7 more than recorded for the 24 typically developing children at 17 months. Of all the different words recorded for the children, 90 percent were said in response to a parent utterance.

After an average of 22 months observing these 5 children with Down syndrome very gradually taking up talking, we began seeing children who appeared prompt-bound, who seemed to say the same thing all the time, and wait to be asked about something different. And still more than half of parent responses followed a child nonword utterance. The more the parents tried to get words from the children, the more often they ended up accepting a nonword utterance.

CONCLUSION AND IMPLICATION

In their efforts to get words from these 5 children with Down syndrome, their parents spent time in joint activities focused on the same topics month after month and prompted a limited range of vocabulary words again and again until the words were over-learned. The pressure was on the parents to make sure the children had the words and concepts the children would need for the tests that would determine the children's educational placement. And the parents' efforts paid off. Eventually all 5 children were talking as much as other members of their families, and all but one of the 5 were fully integrated into public school classrooms.

What was sacrificed was more than a year of experience with conversation. These 5 children with Down syndrome came very late to learning the social dances they would need to make friends in those integrated classrooms. And the data of the 42 typically developing children suggest how difficult catching up is likely to be.

The message from the data of the children with Down syndrome is that environment matters. As we do with the brain, when everything goes right we take the environment for granted, even though we do not really understand how it works. But that understanding is vital. We cannot change the genetics of the children with Down syndrome. We do not need to change the development of language, which is following a typical course. We do not want to change the behavior of the parents, who are doing just what the parents of typically developing children are doing to support and encourage learning to talk. What we can change is the environment, the circumstances of the social dance.

REFERENCES

Bloom, L. 1991. *Language Development from Two to Three.* New York: Cambridge University Press.
Bruner, J. 1983. *Child's Talk: Learning to Use Language.* New York: Norton.
Bullowa, M. (ed.) 1979. *Before Speech.* New York: Cambridge University Press.
Cicchetti, D., and Beeghly, M. 1990. An organizational approach to the study of Down syndrome: Contributions to an integrative theory of development. In *Children with Down Syndrome: A Developmental Perspective*, eds. D. Cicchetti and M. Beeghly. New York: Cambridge University Press.
Dapretto, M., and Bjork, E. L. 2000. The development of word retrieval abilities in the second year and its relation to early vocabulary growth. *Child Development* 71:635–48.
Dromi, E. 1987. *Early Lexical Development.* New York: Cambridge University Press.
Dunn, L. W., and Dunn, L. M. 1981. *Peabody Picture Vocabulary-Revised* (Forms L and M). Circle Pines, MN: American Guidance Service.
Fowler, A. E. 1990. Language abilities in children with Down syndrome. In *Children with Down Syndrome: A Developmental Perspective*, eds. D. Cicchetti and M. Beeghly. New York: Cambridge University Press.
Gelman, R. 1983. Reconsidering the transition from prelinguistic to linguistic communication. In *The Transition from Prelinguistic to Linguistic Communication*, ed. R. M. Golinkoff. Hillsdale, NJ: Lawrence Erlbaum Associates.
Goldfield, B. A., and Reznick, J. S. 1990. Early lexical acquisition: Rate, content, and the vocabulary spurt. *Journal of Child Language* 17:171–83.
Hammill, D. D., and Newcomer, P. L. 1988. *Test of Language Development-2 (TOLD-2): Intermediate (2nd ed.).* Austin, TX: PRO-ED.
Harris, M., Barrett, M., Jones, D., and Brookes, S. 1988. Linguistic input and early word meaning. *Journal of Child Language* 15:77–94.
Hart, B. 1996. The initial growth of expressive vocabulary among children with Down syndrome. *Journal of Early Intervention* 20:211–21.
Hart, B., and Risley, T. R. 1995. *Meaningful Differences in the Everyday Experience of Young American Children.* Baltimore, MD: Paul H. Brookes Publishing.
Hart, B., and Risley, T. R. 1999. *The Social World of Children Learning to Talk.* Baltimore, MD: Paul H. Brookes Publishing.
Locke, J. L. 1996. Why do infants begin to talk? Language as an unintended consequence. *Journal of Child Language* 23:251–68.
Menyuk, P. 1975. Children with language problems: What's the problem? In *Georgetown University Roundtable on Languages and Linguistics*, ed. D. P. Dato. Washington, D. C.: Georgetown University Press.
Miller, J. F. 1987. Language and communication characteristics of children with Down syndrome. In *New Perspectives on Down syndrome*, eds. S. M. Pueschel, C. Tingey, J. E. Rynder, A. C. Crocker, and D. M. Crutcher. Baltimore, MD: Paul H. Brookes Publishing.

Moerk, E. 1989. The LAD was a lady and the tasks were ill-defined. *Developmental Review* 9:21–57.

Nelson, K. 1973. Structure and strategy in learning to talk. *Monographs of the Society for Research in Child Development* 38 (1–2, Serial No. 149).

Roach, M. A., Barratt, M. S., Miller, J. F., and Leavitt, L. A. 1987. The structure of mother-child play: Young children with Down syndrome and typically developing children. *Developmental Psychology* 34:77–87.

Snow, C. E. 1977. The development of conversation between mothers and babies. *Journal of Child Language* 4:1–22.

Snow, C. E. 1986. Conversations with children. In *Language Acquisition: Studies in First Language Development*, eds. P. Fletcher and M. Garman. New York: Cambridge University Press.

Snow, C. E. 1988. The last word: Questions about the emerging lexicon. In *The Emergent Lexicon: The Child's Development of a Linguistic Vocabulary*, eds. M. D. Smith and J. L. Locke. San Diego: Academic Press.

Terman, L. M., and Merrill, M. A. 1960. *Stanford-Binet Intelligence Scale: Manual for the Third Revision, Form L-M.* Boston: Houghton-Mifflin.

Thal, D., Tobias, S., and Morrison, D. 1991. Language and gesture in late talkers: A one-year follow-up. *Journal of Speech and Hearing Research* 34:604–12.

Veneziano, E., and Sinclair, H. 2000. The changing status of 'filler syllables' on the way to grammatical morphemes. *Journal of Child Language* 27:461–500.

Part • II

Language and Hearing

Chapter • 4

Sensitive Periods in the Development of Language of Children Who Are Deaf or Hard of Hearing

Christine Yoshinaga-Itano

Research on the language and speech development of children who are deaf or hard of hearing (D/HH) has provided some evidence that there are sensitive periods of development and that the average child with a significant hearing loss has been unable to demonstrate continuing language development after these periods. Plateaus in language development occur after the age of twelve years for the average child who is deaf or hard of hearing. The literature related to language plateaus is based on the average language scores from cross-sectional databases and therefore, is unable to report longitudinal language growth. Several longitudinal studies have been recently reported and indicate that children with significant hearing loss may actually continue to develop language throughout their school-age years, albeit at very slow and depressed levels when compared to the typical rate of language development.

The language developmental growth rates of children with significant hearing loss were reported by Boothroyd, Geers, and Moog (1991) to be between .43 to .60 of typical development for children between 4 and 18 years of age. One hundred twenty-three children had better pure tone averages (PTA) > 105 dB, and 188 had better pure tone averages between 90 and 104 dB. Geers and Moog (1988) in a study of 44 children between 8 and 14 years of age and 100 students between 16 and 18 years of age, and Blamey et al. (2001) in a study of 47 children with profound loss with cochlear implants and 40 children with severe hearing loss who used conventional hearing aids also reported language developmental rates between .43 and .60 of normal. Svirsky (in press) reported a predictive model of language growth for children who are deaf or hard of hearing, .45 to .50 for pure tone average (PTA) of 90–100 dB and .38 to .41 for PTA 100 dB+.

Historically, children who are deaf or hard of hearing with such slow development (i.e., between 38% to 60% of the typical language development growth pattern) have been reported to plateau at a middle third grade to middle fourth grade reading level (Schildroth and Hotto 1993). These findings may actually be the result of using comparable numbers of children who accelerate in their growth rates and children who decelerate in their growth rate. Combined with children who maintain a steady language growth rate throughout the school-age period, the aggregate result when looking at cross-sectional data leads to a conclusion that children with significant hearing loss plateau in language development, when a plateau is not actually occurring.

Children with hearing loss identified within the first six months of life and who have no secondary disabilities have been found to maintain an average language quotient (LQ = [Language Age/Chronological Age] x 100) of 90 in the first three years of life (Yoshinaga-Itano et al. 1998) and in the first five years of life (Yoshinaga-Itano, Coulter, and Thomson 2000). These results are remarkably similar to the low average language levels described in the Moeller (2000) study of 5-year-old children. These studies are also cross-sectional. However, longitudinal analysis reveals that the vast proportion of children through the first four years of life maintain language growth rates, with only a small percentage either accelerating or decelerating (Stevens 2002). In contrast, the later-identified (LID) children, regardless of degree of hearing loss, had average language quotients of 60 in the first three years of life, which is similar to language growth rates reported in the school-age population (Blamey et al. 2001; Boothroyd, Geers, and Moog 1991; Geers and Moog 1988).

Svirsky et al. (2000) reported significant language delays overall in a cochlear implanted population. However, average age level growth curves over a 6- to 30-month post-implantation period were better than typically found among D/HH children. The best language learners were able to maintain language skills proportionate to chronological age because their language growth curves over this time period were similar to their typically developing peers. Miyamoto, Svirsky, and Robbins (1997) reported accelerated language growth curves over a 6- to 12-month period for children with cochlear implants. However, in the cochlear implant studies, children who are reported to have typical language growth rates for hearing children represent 10% to 20% of the total participants, with only one study reporting on 40% of the total number of children in each study. The language growth rates of the cochlear implant children are reported based upon receptive vocabulary as measured by the Peabody Picture Vocabulary Test (PPVT).

Several important questions arise. The percentage of children in the total population of children with significant hearing loss who are able to accelerate their language growth rates and the variables that predict membership in this group of accelerators are very important. It is also critically important to determine whether accelerated growth patterns can be maintained over longer periods of time in order to reduce the significant delays in language and literacy development typically noted in the deaf and hard of hearing population. Additionally, other language measures in addition to the PPVT need to be used to identify language growth rates in the school-age population. Because almost all of the longitudinal studies rely upon a single measure of language growth, a more comprehensive picture of language will provide valuable information about how children with significant hearing loss learn.

Previous research studies initially focused on children with profound hearing loss, and language growth curves of children with severe hearing loss have only recently been available. Information on the subgroup of children with significant, but less severe, hearing loss is rare. Two studies conducted with this population found that the means of all subgroups of children (three groups by degree of hearing loss and two groups by age [< 12 yrs, > 12 yrs]) on the Peabody Picture Vocabulary Test-Revised fell below the norms for the test. However, only 11 of the 40 children were aided before age 4 and only 1 was aided before 2 years of age (Davis et al. 1986; Shepard et al. 1981). Because 50% of the children identified through universal newborn hearing screening (UNHS) programs have mild to moderate hearing loss (Dalzell et al. 2000), it may be possible to identify language growth rates among children with hearing loss in the mild to moderate range.

Studies of children who are deaf or hard of hearing could have significant implications for discussions regarding sensitive periods of development. It is possible that sensitive periods of development exist among this population of children because they have failed to master specific language skills by a critical age level due to lack of full access to a comprehensive language model, thereby making it very difficult to develop language beyond certain levels. Alternately, there is evidence that certain bursts of development, such as vocabulary bursts (at the two year age level), if delayed beyond a certain age level, fail to occur, resulting in a deceleration of language growth rate because the child continues developing language in a linear pattern rather than evidencing periods of significant language bursts.

SENSITIVE PERIODS OF DEVELOPMENT/ WINDOWS OF OPPORTUNITY FOR DEVELOPMENT

A sensitive period for language development during the first six months of life has been identified through the research generated from the first six years of the Colorado project (Yoshinaga-Itano et al. 1998; Mayne et al. 2000; Mayne et al. 2000; Yoshinaga-Itano and Apuzzo 1998a and b). Among the later-identified children, 16% to 25% are able to maintain language growth similar to the early-identified children. Those later-identified children with the highest cognitive levels from families with the highest socio-economic levels and the mildest hearing losses are most likely to be successful in their language development.

Early identification/intervention

Yoshinaga-Itano et al. (1998) in a study of 150 deaf and hard-of-hearing infants and toddlers found significantly higher language development among children identified with hearing loss and placed into intervention by 6 months of age. The first 6 months of life appear to represent a particularly sensitive period in early language development. Access to language during this period provides an opportunity for children with significant hearing loss to develop language skills that are slightly depressed from the mean language of children with normal hearing (low average), but within the normal developmental continuum.

Participants. We studied 72 children between the ages of 12 to 36 months who were identified with hearing loss prior to 6 months of age. Twenty-five of these children were participants in the Apuzzo and Yoshinaga-Itano (1995) study of children identified through the high risk registry. Forty-seven children identified through universal newborn hearing screening (UNHS) were included in this study. They represented approximately 70% of the eligible participants identified after UNHS programs had been initiated in Colorado from 1992 through 1996.

The 72 early-identified participants (EID) were matched to 78 later-identified participants from an existing database of over 350 infants and toddlers. The participants were matched according to degree of hearing loss, age at time of testing, gender, ethnicity, socio-economic status (maternal level of education and Medicaid status), presence/absence of secondary disabilities, and non-verbal symbolic play development.

Early-identified children had some characteristics that made matching difficult. Non-verbal symbolic play development of the early-identified children was slightly higher than in the later-identified children. Although this difference was not significant, symbolic play development was used as a covariance variable. Additionally, early-identified children with milder hearing losses can be identified through UNHS and these children, if missed at birth, are frequently not identified until school-age unless they also have additional disabilities. No significant differences by any of the matching variables were found. No significant differences in the language quotients ([Language Age/Chronological Age] x 100) were found for children identified between birth through two months, three and four months, and five and six months. (See figure 1.)

Early-identified (0–6 mo.) children had significantly higher language quotients (LQ = 80) than 1) children identified between 7–12 months (LQ = 59), 2) between 13–18 months (LQ = 60), 3) between 19–24 months (LQ = 60), and 4) between 25–34 months of age (LQ = 56). Forty percent of these children had multiple disabilities. (See figure 2.)

This sensitive period is applicable within the first 36 months of life to all groups by degree of hearing loss, both groups by method of communication, both genders, children with hearing loss only and those with additional disabilities, all groups by ethnic background and by socio-economic status, and at each age level tested (12, 18, 24, 30, 36 months of age).

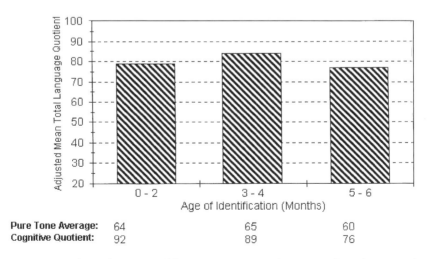

Figure 1   Adjusted mean total language quotients for groups based on age of identification of hearing loss. This graph includes only children in the early identification category.

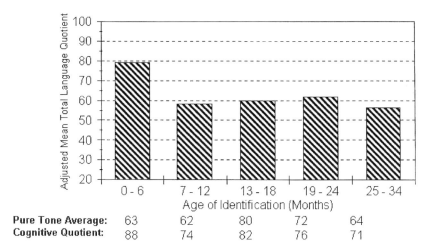

Age of Identification (Months)	0 - 6	7 - 12	13 - 18	19 - 24	25 - 34
Pure Tone Average:	63	62	80	72	64
Cognitive Quotient:	88	74	82	76	71

Figure 2   Adjusted mean total language quotients for groups based on age of identification of hearing loss. (Reprinted with permission from *Pediatrics*, Yoshinaga-Itano, Sedey, Coulter, and Mehl 1998 102(5):1161–71)

Age at Testing.   The language advantage that characterized the early-identified group was present at all test ages. No developmental effects were found. Early-identified children had significantly higher language development than LID children when tested at 12 months, 18 months, 24 months, 30 months and 36 months of age. Thus, the impact of early identification and intervention can be observed at 12 months of age and throughout the first 3 years of life. These results are similar to those obtained by Apuzzo and Yoshinaga-Itano (1995). (See figure 3.)

Mode of Communication.   Early identification was associated with better language development for all families regardless of method of communication. Early-identified children obtained higher language scores than LID children regardless of whether the families chose oral methods of communication or communication with sign language. Moeller (2000) also found that method of communication was not related to language outcomes of either early-identified or later-identified children. (See figure 4.)

Ethnicity.   Both EID children from Caucasian ethnic backgrounds and other ethnic backgrounds (predominantly Latino) evidenced significantly better language development than their LID counterparts. The historical literature in deafness contains developmental data indicating that children from ethnic minority backgrounds have significantly lower academic and language achievement than those children from ethnic majority backgrounds. The Colorado

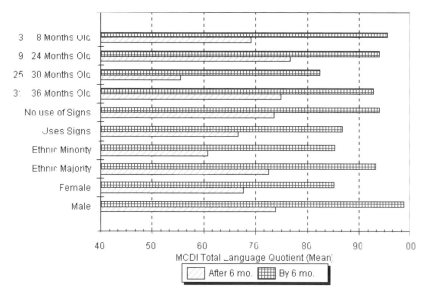

Figure 3   Early identification effect by age, mode of communication, ethnicity, and gender (Reprinted with permission from *Pediatrics*, Yoshinaga-Itano, Sedey, Coulter, and Mehl 1998 102(5):1161–71)

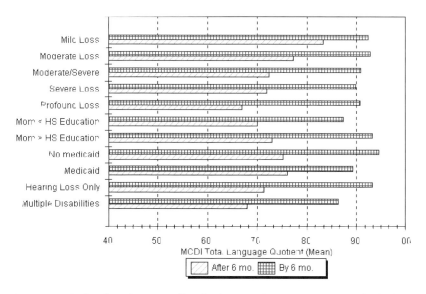

Figure 4   Early identification effect by hearing loss, maternal level of education, Medicaid status, and presence/absence of additional disabilities. (Reprinted with permission from *Pediatrics*, Yoshinaga-Itano, Sedey, Coulter, and Mehl 1998 102(5):1161–71)

population of deaf and hard of hearing children is approximately 75% Caucasian (non-Hispanic), 20% to 25% Hispanic, and 1% to 5% other (Asian, Native American, African American). Ethnicity has been found to be highly related to reading outcomes among deaf and hard of hearing school-aged children (Office of Demographic Studies). (See figure 4.)

Degree of Hearing loss.   Early-identified children with mild, moderate, moderately severe, severe, and profound hearing loss had similar language development. Early-identified children with hearing loss and no additional disabilities, regardless of degree of hearing loss, had language development that was 90% of their chronological age. When children were identified later and had no secondary disabilities, their language development was significantly better with better hearing, and on average, the later-identified children had language development which was 60% to 70% of their chronological age. Moeller (2000) also found that degree of hearing loss failed to predict language outcomes of the children in her study. (See figure 3.)

Socio-economic status.   Early-identified children from families with low, middle, or high socio-economic status, as measured by maternal level of education and qualification for Medicaid, had better language development than children who were identified later regardless of socio-economic level. These findings differ somewhat from the language development of children with normal hearing. Socio-economic variables, particularly maternal level of education, have been associated with better language development among children without disabilities. In the first three years of life, higher socio-economic status does not appear to be associated with better language development in this Colorado sample of deaf and hard of hearing children. These findings may indicate that intervention techniques that characterize the home intervention program provide an equalizing effect to the normal advantages associated with greater income and higher education. This sample contained a significant number of families with very low incomes and low educational levels. (See figure 3.)

Presence of Additional Disability.   A significant proportion of children who are deaf or hard of hearing have secondary disabilities. The language advantage associated with early identification/intervention was found for both children with hearing loss only and children with secondary disabilities.

As mentioned previously, when identified early, children with secondary disabilities had non-verbal symbolic play development that was similar to their language development, while children who were identified later with secondary disabilities had ten to fifteen point discrepancies between their non-verbal cognitive development and their language development. (See figure 3.)

Gender.   Significant differences in the language quotients of boys and girls were found with a surprising result. Young boys had significantly higher language quotients than girls, a finding that is in direct contrast to research on the typical development of infants and toddlers with normal hearing. Raw scores of the two groups were not significantly different, but the Minnesota Child Development Inventory adjusts for previously found gender differences and provides a higher language quotient for a boy with the same raw score as a girl. (See figure 4.)

Yoshinaga-Itano, Coulter, and Thomson (2000) also reported that the effect of age of identification extended to children who were 60 months of age. Stevens (2002) has found that the impact of age of identification/intervention remains at least until 48 months of life in a longitudinal sample, but there is some indication that the nature of the relationship begins to change from a dichotomous (before 6 months/after 6 months) to a continuous relationship (earlier is better).

Language development within the normal range of development

On average, children with early identification/intervention with no additional disabilities were found to have language development in the low range of normal language development at all testing ages through the first three years of life when using both a general measure of language and a specific measure of vocabulary. In a study of the effectiveness of screening for hearing loss (N = 294), 80% of the children with hearing loss and no secondary disabilities born in hospitals that had instituted a newborn hearing screening program achieved language development at a quotient of 80 or higher (Yoshinaga-Itano, Coulter, and Thomson 2000). Moeller (2000) found similar language functioning among her early-identified children at five years of age. This finding is in contrast to previous reports that children with significant hearing loss typically demonstrate language development at levels between the 1st and 10th percentile (Blamey et al. 2001).

Impact of time in intervention in the first three years of life

There was a non-significant relationship (r = .08) between the time in intervention and the language developmental quotient among the late identified/intervened group, indicating that within the first 3 years of life, amount of time in intervention did not significantly reduce the relationship between language delay and chronological age (Yoshinaga-Itano et al. 1998). However, data analysis reveals an impact of age of identification more in a continuous linear fashion than a dichotomous threshold after the age of 3 years, indicating that effects of time in intervention may begin to emerge after 3 years of age. These data are consistent with the findings of Moeller (2000) on a group of 5-year-old children with hearing loss.

Language quotients comparable to cognitive quotients

The early-identified/early intervention (EID) children maintained language development similar to their non-verbal cognitive symbolic play development, while later-identified/intervention (LID) children evidenced greater than a 20 point discrepancy between non-verbal cognitive development and language development. Cognitive symbolic play quotients and language quotients were similar for early-identified children (Yoshinaga-Itano et al. 1998). Note in figures 5 and 6 that the EID groups, represented with solid bars, have no more than a five point discrepancy between non-verbal symbolic play and expressive language. The LID group has an average 20 to 25 point discrepancy for children with hearing loss only, represented by the hatched bars.

Discrepancies between non-verbal intelligence quotients and verbal intelligence quotients among the school-aged population who are D/HH have been reported, even among the most educationally successful students. It is interesting to note that 20 point discrepancies are commonly found among college-bound children with significant hearing loss, while discrepancies as great as 40 points in the non-college bound children have been reported (Geers, and Moog 1989; Levitt et al. 1987, Osberger et al. 1986).

Early-identification and cognitive status. Early-identified children with secondary disabilities had remarkable similarities in lan-

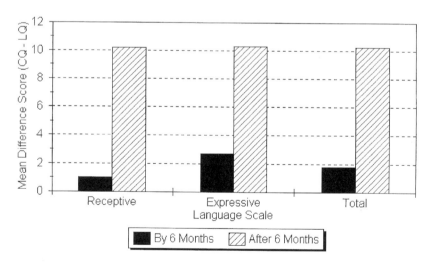

Figure 5   Discrepancy between cognitive quotient and language quotient by age of identification of hearing loss for children with low cognition. (Reprinted with permission from *Pediatrics*, Yoshinaga-Itano, Sedey, Coulter, and Mehl 1998 102(5):1161–71)

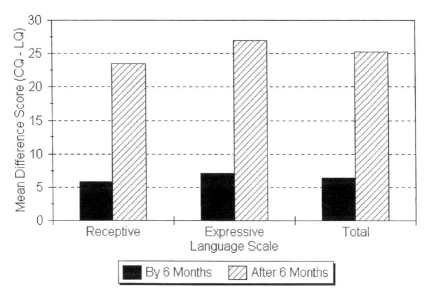

Figure 6   Discrepancy between cognitive quotient and language quotient by age of identification of hearing loss for children with normal cognition. (Reprinted with permission from *Pediatrics*, Yoshinaga-Itano, Sedey, Coulter, and Mehl 1998 102(5):1161–71)

guage quotients to LID children with hearing loss only. Both groups were significantly different from EID children with hearing loss only, but not from one another. The LID children with additional disabilities had the lowest language development. Later identification of hearing loss with later onset of intervention services for those children with hearing loss and no secondary disabilities results in language development more similar to multiply disabled children who are early-identified (Yoshinaga-Itano et al. 1998). (See figure 7.)

EARLY IDENTIFICATION/INTERVENTION AND VOCABULARY DEVELOPMENT

Vocabulary development

Children with normal hearing compared to children with EID hearing loss.   Early-identified children with significant hearing loss who had normal cognitive development had vocabulary development that was approximately 25 percentile lower than children without hearing loss. The EID children ranged in vocabulary scores from the 10th percentile of the normal distribution through the 90th percentile.

Children with LID hearing loss compared to EID children and children with normal hearing.   Mayne et al. (2000), in a study of 112

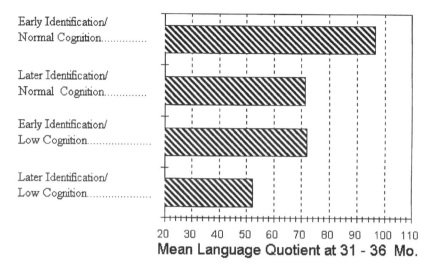

Figure 7   Mean total language quotient scores at 31 to 36 months by age of identification of hearing loss and cognition. (Reprinted with permission from *Pediatrics*, Yoshinaga-Itano, Sedey, Coulter, and Mehl 1998 102(5):1161–71)

infants and toddlers with significant hearing loss, using multiple regression analyses with a block design, found that the situation comprehension quotient from the Minnesota Child Development Inventory and age of identification of hearing loss predicted vocabulary development. Gender, race/ethnicity, socio-economic status, degree of hearing loss, mode of communication, and age at testing, all failed to significantly predict expressive vocabulary development. (See figures 8 and 9.)

The vocabulary scores of over 300 children with significant hearing loss were plotted. Later-identified children with significant hearing loss had vocabulary development that was 50 percentile lower than children without hearing loss during the first 36 months of life. Thus, the top 25th percentile of the later-identified children fell at the bottom 25 percentile of the distribution for children with normal hearing. For children with early-identified hearing loss and early intervention, the top 25th percentile of the later-identified children's vocabulary development fell at the bottom 25th percentile of the distribution of normally hearing children. Seventy five percent of the LID fell below the 10th percentile of the distribution for normally hearing children.

The rapid development of expressive vocabulary levels in the third year of life present interesting dilemmas for the early intervention provider. As will be discussed in the following section, only the

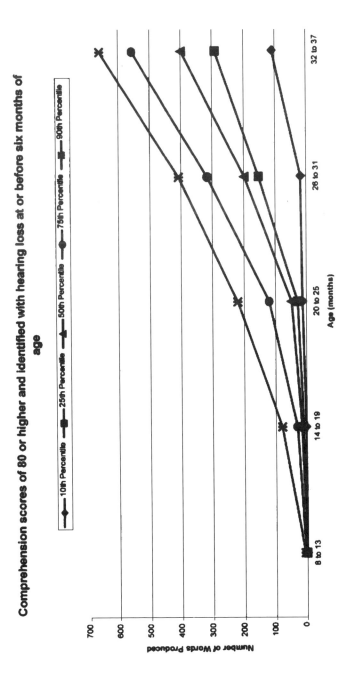

Figure 8   Expressive language quotients of children who are deaf or hard of hearing with Situation Comprehension Quotients 80 or higher and identified with hearing loss prior to six months of age. (Reprinted with permission from the *Volta Review*.)

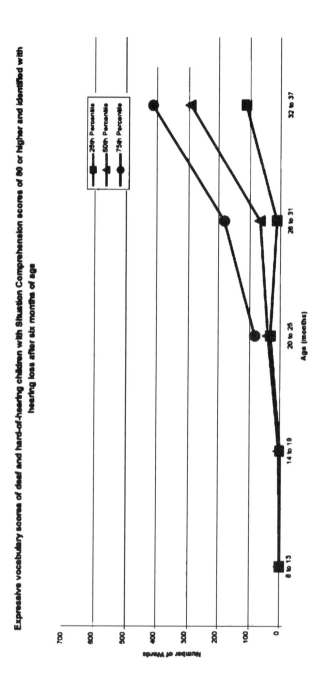

Figure 9   Expressive language scores of children who are deaf or hard of hearing with Situation Comprehension Quotients 80 or higher and identified with hearing loss after six months of age. (Reprinted with permission from the *Volta Review*.)

children with mild hearing loss begin to develop speech repertoires similar to their hearing peers at the age of greatest vocabulary growth. Even early-identified children with mild hearing loss may be sufficiently delayed in speech development to affect their intelligibility. Children with moderate through profound hearing loss, while developing intelligible speech by 5 years of age, have unintelligible utterances to naïve listeners until about 60 months of age. Thus, individuals teaching sign language to families must have strong skills in order to facilitate family sign language development so that the families have thousands of words in their sign lexicon in the child's preschool years. The child with hearing loss will have significantly better comprehension than speech intelligibility when communicating orally. Early intervention providers must be careful to ensure that this imbalance does not have a negative impact on the social-emotional development of the child, because difficulty in communicating can lead to behavior such as outbursts or tantrums.

Plateau in speech intelligibility. A second plateau that has been reported in the literature is the failure to demonstrate average developmental speech intelligibility gains after the age of 8 years (Jensema, Karchmer, and Trybus 1978).

Speech development

The development of speech appears to maintain a much longer window of development than the development of other aspects of language. Early-identified children with hearing loss of any degree have speech that differs significantly from children with normal hearing. This difference continues at least through the first 2 years of life (Wallace, Menn, and Yoshinaga-Itano 2000; Obenchain, Menn, and Yoshinaga-Itano 2000). In a longitudinal study of 20 infants examined at three age levels: between 5 and 13 months, between 2 and 5 years and between 5 and 10 years, Mean Babble Level was not found to be significantly related to speech development (Wallace et al. 2000). Some of the children with very simple babble production developed intelligible speech, whereas some of the children with more complex early babble production were not speaking intelligibly by early elementary school. Children with no babble in the first year of life could develop intelligible speech both between 2 and 5 years of age and between 5 and 10 years.

In a longitudinal study of 19 children who are deaf or hard of hearing, speech and language characteristics present at 16 to 23 months of age distinguished children who developed intelligible speech by 36 months. Children with a high frequency of vocal utterances, a relatively high proportion of vocal utterances that included intelligible true words, a relatively large lexical inventory (more than nine spoken words), a large consonant inventory, a high percentage of rising tones, a high percentage of intonational utterances (speech and/or jargon), a large percentage of syllables containing consonants, and a tendency to show intention through the use of gesture even in utterances with no semantic content were the most likely to develop intelligible speech by 36 months.

Children with mild hearing losses master the articulation of spoken English by 3 years of age, but children with moderate and severe hearing losses show most of their speech development between 3 and 5 years of age. (See figures 11 and 13.) Children with later-identified hearing losses do equally well in their speech development as children with early-identified hearing loss when language development is comparable (Yoshinaga-Itano and Sedey 2000). Significant predictors of speech intelligibility and phonetic inventory included the child's age, expressive language ability, degree of hearing loss, mode of communication, and, for some of the speech variables, the presence of additional disabilities. (See figures 10 and 12).

Early identification and speech development. Apuzzo and Yoshinaga-Itano (1995) found significantly better speech production of early-identified children when compared to later-identified children. Yoshinaga-Itano, Coulter, and Thomson (2000) found that children with hearing loss born in hospitals with UNHS programs had

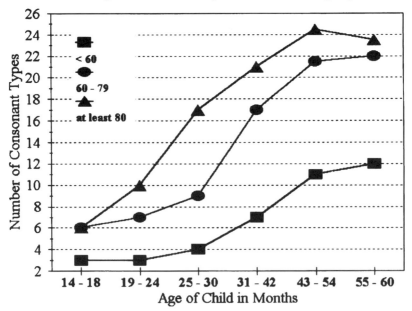

Figure 10   Number of consonant types by age and expressive language quotient. (Reprinted with permission from the *Volta Review*.)

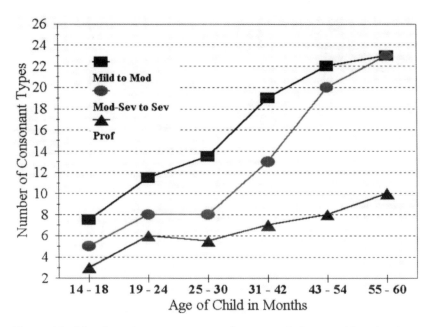

Figure 11   Number of consonant types by age and degree of hearing loss. (Reprinted with permission from the *Volta Review*.)

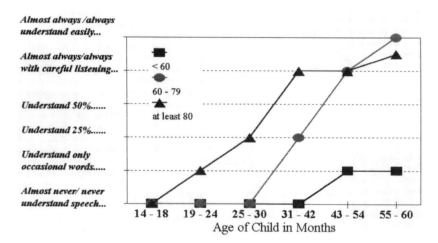

Figure 12   Speech intelligibility by age and expressive language quotient. (Reprinted with permission from the *Volta Review*.)

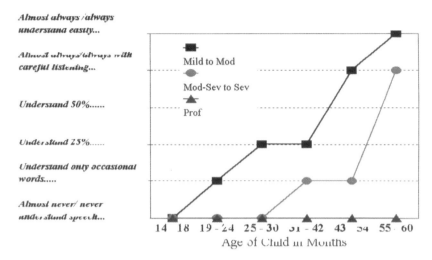

Figure 13   Speech intelligibility by age and degree of hearing loss. (Reprinted with permission from the *Volta Review*.)

significantly better speech intelligibility, and number of consonants in spontaneous speech samples.

Cognitive development

Research completed to date indicates that language development, when age is accounted for by developmental quotients, is highly re-lated to the development of symbolic play, situation comprehension, early identification of the hearing loss, and emotional availability of the parent (Mayne et al. 2000a and b; Pipp-Siegel 2000; Yoshinaga-Itano et al. 1998). Non-verbal cognitive development has not been highly predictive of language or academic achievement within the school-age period and accounted for only about 9% of the variance in academic achievement (Levitt, McGarr, and Geffner 1987; Geers and Moog 1989). Thus, continuation of the longitudinal study may allow us to examine whether this relationship established in infancy and the toddler years prevails throughout the early childhood period.

Autosymbolic play, age of identification, and symbolic substitu-tion accounted for 41.8% of the variance in expressive language of in-fants and toddlers who are D/HH (Snyder and Yoshinaga-Itano 1999). When the Play Assessment Questionnaire was used as an index of symbolic play, the Symbolic Play Quotient accounted for 44% of the variance in productive vocabulary, with an additional 3% of the vari-ance accounted for by age of identification (Yoshinaga-Itano and Snyder 1999). Mayne et al. (2000) reported that 56% of the variance in expressive vocabulary scores of children birth through 37 months of age was accounted for by child's age, age of identification, Situation-Comprehension quotient of the Minnesota Child Development Inventory, and whether the child had additional medical conditions.

Social Emotional Development and Family Stress

Another focus of the 1994–2000 research project was the social-emotional development of D/HH infants and preschoolers. Emotional availability was used as a measure of attachment and bonding. In general, the higher the language skill, the better the reciprocal emotional availability of mother and child. Pressman et al. (1999) reported that emotional availability (e.g., maternal sensitivity to infants and infant responsiveness to mothers) when infants were 2 years of age predicted gain in expressive language when the infants were 3 years. Pressman et al. (2000) reported that emotional availability made significantly greater positive predictions of child language gain for children who are D/HH than for children with normal hearing. The language of children who are deaf or hard of hearing seems to be more responsive to greater maternal sensitivity.

Emotional availability was related to the number of times hearing mothers touched their hearing children, with more touches related to higher maternal intrusiveness scores. No relationship, however, was seen between touch and emotional availability in hearing mothers of D/HH children (Pipp-Siegel et al. 2000). The authors concluded that touch was used as a means of communication for dyads with a D/HH infant and so was unrelated to emotional availability, but was seen as intrusive for dyads with hearing infants.

A third study examined self-recognition and self-description/evaluation in a group of 53 14- to 40-month-old children who are D/HH. Self recognition of D/HH children was similar to typically developing children. Self-description/evaluation increased significantly as the child aged and as the age of identification decreased. These relationships were mediated by expressive language (Pressman 2000).

Finally, predictors of maternal stress were assessed (Pipp-Siegel, Sedey, and Yoshinaga-Itano 2001). Stress levels were measured in three domains using the short form of the Parental Stress Index (PSI) (Abidin 1997). Mothers in this study demonstrated significantly less Parental Distress on the PSI than a normative, hearing group, although this difference was quite small. No significant differences between the mothers of children who are D/HH and mothers of hearing children was found for the Dysfunctional Parent-Child Interactions or the Difficult Child subscales. Mothers who perceived their daily hassles as more intense also obtained higher stress ratings on all three subscales. Additional predictors of the Parental Distress subscale were frequency of hassles, social support, and annual family income.

Increased stress on the Dysfunctional Parent-Child Interaction sub-scale was predicted by children who had disabilities in addition to hearing loss, more delayed language relative to their chronological age, and less severe degrees of hearing loss. No additional significant predictors were obtained for the Difficult Child subscale. When all measured variables were controlled for, characteristics that did not predict maternal stress on any of the three subscales included the child's gender, ethnicity, age of identification, mode of communication used, months between age of identification and child age at time of observation, and maternal education.

The age of identification of hearing loss in the first 6 months of life is highly related to language development and personal-social de-velopment. Early-identified children had higher personal-social devel-opment. Later-identified children with mild hearing loss had lower personal-social development than EID children with all degrees of hearing loss and LID children with moderate, severe, and profound hearing loss. Personal-social development, similar to language devel-opment, is highly related to symbolic play, presence of additional medical conditions, and the discrepancy between language and chronological age (Yoshinaga-Itano and Abdala de Uzcategui 2001; Downs and Yoshinaga-Itano 1999).

EARLY IDENTIFICATION/INTERVENTION AND SOCIAL-EMOTIONAL DEVELOPMENT

Personal-Social Development

Early-identified children had significantly higher personal-social skill development than children whose hearing losses were identified later. Children with mild hearing loss evidenced the greatest discrepancy between early-identified and later-identified children. The later-identified children with mild hearing loss had poorer personal-social skills than later-identified children with moderate to profound hear-ing loss. Gender, degree of hearing loss, socio-economic status, race/ethnicity, mode of communication, and age at testing failed to predict personal-social development. (See figure 14.)

Self-Development

Pressman (2000) examined the self-recognition and self-description/ evaluation in a group of 53 14- to 40-month old children who were deaf or hard of hearing using the Stipek, Gralinski, and Kopp (1990) Self-Concept Questionnaire. Self-recognition of children who are deaf or hard of hearing was similar for children of the same ages who had normal hearing. Self-recognition development increases significantly with age from 14 to 40 months and the majority of self-recognition

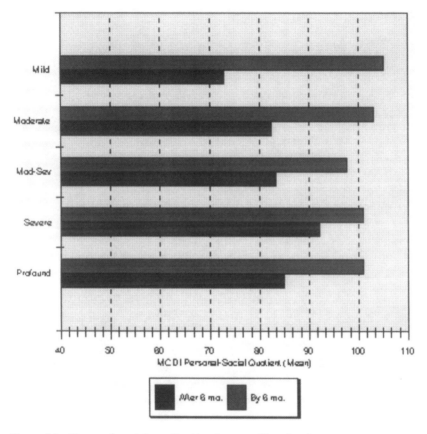

Figure 14   Personal-social quotient by degree of hearing loss.

items were passed before the majority of self-description/evaluation. Expressive language development completed accounted for the relationship between self-recognition and age. Self-description/ evaluation increased significantly with age. However, the later the age of identification, the lower the self-description/evaluation scores even when child and family characteristics were controlled. The relationship between self description/evaluation, age, and age of identification were partially accounted for by expressive language, but age of identification contributed to the development of self-description/ evaluation over and above expressive language ability.

Even at very early ages in development, expressive language is highly related to self-concept development. Although some aspects of self-concept development are not highly related to language development, a significant component of self-development at this age appears to be dependent upon language.

SUMMARY

Yoshinaga-Itano et al. (1998) were able to study a cohort of 150 children, 72 EID and 78 LID. They reported significantly higher language developmental outcomes of the EID children as compared to the 78 LID children matched on a variety of demographic variables (symbolic play development, degree of hearing loss, gender, ethnicity, maternal educational level, presence/absence of secondary disability, Medicaid eligibility, mode of communication, and age at testing). These findings were replicated by Mayne et al. (2000) in a study of expressive vocabulary. Moeller (2000) reported significantly higher language outcomes at age 5 years for children with significant hearing loss whose intervention was initiated by 11 months of age. Yoshinaga-Itano, Coulter, and Thomson (2000) reported significantly higher language outcomes from 12 months through 60 months for a group of children with hearing loss born in hospitals with UNHS programs. Moeller (2000), Yoshinaga-Itano et al. (1998), and Yoshinaga-Itano et al. (2000) report that children with early-identified hearing loss who receive early intervention attain language development at low average levels in the first five years of life if they have no secondary disabilities.

Thus, these sensitive periods of language development appear to be related to environmental factors and access to information. Earlier identification and intervention provide the opportunity for children with significant hearing loss to access the same type and amount of language information available to children with normal hearing.

ACKNOWLEDGMENTS

Research summarized in this chapter was funded by the National Institutes of Health, N01-4-2141, the Office of Education, Maternal and Child Health, the Colorado Department of Public Health and Environment, the Colorado Department of Education, and the University of Colorado-Boulder.

REFERENCES

Abidin, R. R. 1997. *Parental Stress Index, 3rd Edition.* Odessa, FL: Psychological Assessment Resources.

Apuzzo, M., and Yoshinaga-Itano, C. 1995. Early identification of infants with significant hearing loss and the Minnesota Child Development Inventory. *Seminars in Hearing* 16(2):124–39.

Blamey, P. J., Sarant, J. Z., Paatsch, L. E., Barry, J. G., Bow, C. P., Wales, R. J., Wright, M., Psarros, C., Rattigan, K., and Tooher, R. 2001. Relationships among speech perception, production, language, hearing loss, and age in children with impaired hearing. *Journal of Speech, Language, and Hearing Research* 44(2):264–85.

Boothroyd, A., Geers, A. E., and Moog, J. S. 1991. Practical implications of cochlear implants in children. *Ear and Hearing* 12:81S–89S.

Dalzell, L., Orlando, M., MacDonald, M., Berg, A., Bradley, M., Cacace, A., Campbell, D., DeCristofaro, J., Gravel, J., Greenberg, E., Gross, S., Pinheiro, J., Regan, J., Spivak, L., Stevens, F., and Prieve, B. 2000. The New York State universal newborn hearing screening demonstration project: Ages of hearing loss identification, hearing aid fitting, and enrollment in early intervention. *Ear and Hearing* 21(2):188–30.

Davis, J. M., Elfenbein, J., Schum, R., and Bentler, R. A. 1986. Effects of mild and moderate hearing impairments on language, educational, and psychosocial behavior of children. *Journal of Speech and Hearing Disorders* 51:53–62.

Downs, M. P., and Yoshinaga-Itano, C. 1999. The efficacy of early identification and intervention for the child with hearing impairment. In *Pediatric Clinics of North America* 46:79–87, eds. N. J. Roizen and A. O. Diefendorf.

Geers, A. E., and Moog, J. S. 1988. Predicting long-term benefits from single-channel cochlear implants in profoundly hearing-impaired children. *American Journal of Otology* 9:169–76.

Geers, A., and Moog, J. 1989. Factors predictive of the development of literacy in profoundly hearing-impaired adolescents. *The Volta Review* 91:69–86.

Jensema, C. J., Karchmer, M. A., and Trybus, R. J. 1978. The rates speech intelligibility of hearing-impaired children: Basic relationships. Washington, DC: Gallaudet College Office of Demographic Studies.

Levitt, H., McGarr, N., and Geffner, D. 1987. Monographs of the American Speech, Language and Hearing Association, 26.

Mayne, A., Yoshinaga-Itano, C., and Sedey, A. 2000. Receptive vocabulary development of infants and toddlers who are deaf or hard of hearing. In *Language, Speech and Social-Emotional Development of Children Who Are Deaf and Hard-of-Hearing: The Early Years*, eds. C. Yoshinaga-Itano and A. L. Sedey. *The Volta Review* 100:29–52.

Mayne, A. M., Yoshinaga-Itano, C., Sedey, A. L., and Carey, A. 2000. Expressive vocabulary development of infants and toddlers who are deaf or hard of hearing. *The Volta Review* 100(5):1–28.

Miyamoto, R. T., Svirsky, M. A., and Robbins, A. M. 1997. Enhancement of expressive language in prelingually deaf children with cochlear implants. *Acta Otolaryngology* (Stockholm) 117(2):154–57.

Moeller, M. P. 2000. Early intervention and language development in children who are deaf and hard of hearing. *Pediatrics* 106:E43.

Obenchain, P., Menn, L., and Yoshinaga-Itano, C. 2000. Can speech development at thirty-six months in children with hearing loss be predicted from information available in the second year of life? In *Language, Speech and Social-Emotional Development of Children Who Are Deaf and Hard-of-Hearing: The Early Years*, eds. C. Yoshinaga-Itano and A. L. Sedey. *The Volta Review* 100:149–80.

Osberger, M. J., Moeller, M. P., Eccarius, M., Robbins, A. M., and Johnson, D. 1986. Language and learning skills of hearing-impaired students. Expressive language skills. *ASHA Monograph* (1986 Mar) 23:54–65.

Pipp-Siegel, S., Sedey, A. L., and Yoshinaga-Itano, C., 2001. Predictors of parental stress in mothers of young children with hearing loss. *Journal of Deaf Studies and Deaf Education* 7(10):1–17.

Pipp-Siegel, S. 2000. Resolution of grief of parents with young children with hearing loss. Unpublished manuscript. Boulder, CO: University of Colorado.

Pipp-Siegel, S., Blair, N., Deas, A., Pressman, L., and Yoshinaga-Itano, C. 2000. Touch and emotional availability in hearing and deaf or hard-of-hearing toddlers and their hearing mothers. In *Language, Speech and Social-Emotional Development of Children Who Are Deaf and Hard-of-Hearing: The Early Years*, eds. C. Yoshinaga-Itano and A. L. Sedey. *The Volta Review* 100:179–98.

Pressman, L. 2000. Early Self-Development in Children with Hearing Loss. Unpublished doctoral dissertation. Boulder, CO: University of Colorado.

Pressman, L., Pipp-Siegel, S., Yoshinaga-Itano, C., and Deas, A. 1999. The relation of sensitivity to child expressive language gain in deaf and hard-of-hearing children whose caregivers are hearing. *The Journal of Deaf Studies and Deaf Education* 4(4):294–304.

Pressman, L., Pipp-Siegel, S., Yoshinaga-Itano, C., Kubicek, L., and Emde, R. N. 2000. A comparison of the links between emotional availability and language gain in young children with and without hearing loss. In *Language, Speech and Social-Emotional Development of Deaf and Hard-of-Hearing Children: The Early Years*, eds. C. Yoshinaga-Itano and A. Sedey. *The Volta Review*, 100(5)

Schildroth, A. N., and Hotto, S. A. 1993. Annual survey of hearing-impaired children and youth, 1991–92 school year. *American Annals of the Deaf* 138:163–71.

Shepard, N. T., Davis, J. M., Gorga, M. P., and Stelmachowicz, P. G. 1981. Characteristics of hearing-impaired children in the public schools: Part I—demographic data. *Journal of Speech and Hearing Disorders* 46(2):123–9.

Siegel, S. 2000. Resolution of grief of parents with young children with hearing loss. Unpublished manuscript. Boulder, CO: University of Colorado.

Snyder, L., and Yoshinaga-Itano, C. 1999. Specific play behaviors and the development of communication in children with hearing loss. *The Volta Review* 100(3):165–85 .

Stevens, C. 2002. Stability of language development from 36 to 48 months in children who are deaf or hard of hearing. Unpublished master's thesis, University of Colorado, Boulder.

Stipek, D. J., Gralinski, H., and Kopp, C. B. 1990. Self-concept development in the toddler years. *Developmental Psychology* 26:972–77.

Svirsky, M. A. in press. Language development in children with profound and prelingual hearing loss, without cochlear implants. *Language* 185: 99–100.

Svirsky, M. A., Robbins, A. M., Kirk, K. I., Pisoni, D. B., and Miyamoto, R. T. 2000. Language development in profoundly deaf children with cochlear implants. *Psychological Science* 11(2):153–58.

Wallace, V., Menn, L., and Yoshinaga-Itano, C. 2000. Is babble the gateway to speech for all children? A longitudinal study of deaf and hard-of-hearing infants. In *Language, Speech and Social-Emotional Development of Deaf and Hard-of-Hearing Children: The Early Years*, eds. C. Yoshinaga and A. Sedey, *The Volta Review* 100(5).

Yoshinaga-Itano, C., and Abdala de Uzcategui, C. 2001. Early identification and social emotional factors of children with hearing loss and children screened for hearing loss. In *Early Childhood Deafness*, eds. E. Kurtzer-White and D. Luterman. Baltimore: York Press.

Yoshinaga-Itano, C., and Apuzzo, M. 1998a. Identification of hearing loss after 18 months is not early enough. *American Annals of the Deaf* 143:380–87.

Yoshinaga-Itano, C., and Apuzzo, M. 1998b. The development of deaf and hard-of-hearing children identified early through the high risk registry. *American Annals of the Deaf* 143:416–24.

Yoshinaga-Itano, C., Coulter, D., and Thomson, V. 2000. The Colorado Newborn Hearing Screening Project: Effects on speech and language development for children with hearing loss. *Journal of Perinatology* 20(8–2): S132–37.

Yoshinaga-Itano, C., Sedey, A., Coulter, D., and Mehl, A. 1998. Language of early- and later-identified children with hearing loss. *Pediatrics* 102(5): 1161–71.

Yoshinaga-Itano, C., and Sedey, A. 2000. Speech development of deaf and hard-of-hearing children in early childhood: Interrelationships with Language and Hearing. In *Language, Speech and Social-Emotional Development of Deaf and Hard-of-hearing Children: The Early Years*, C. Yoshinaga-Itano and A. Sedey. *The Volta Review* 100(5).

Yoshinaga-Itano, C., and Snyder, L. 1999. The relationship of language and symbolic play in deaf and hard-of-hearing children. *The Volta Review* 100(3):135–64.

Chapter • 5

Otitis Media: Is there a Relationship to Language Development?

Robert J. Ruben

Language is a biological function that differs from traditionally accessed biological functions in the degree to which it depends both on the intrinsic nature of the individual and the ways in which the environment and culture have shaped a particular central nervous system. Language is the interface between biology and culture. Thus, to address the question of the relationship of otitis media and language, one must consider the many intrinsic and extrinsic factors that contribute to development of a person's language. First we will look briefly at the historical background of the question; then we will examine some mechanisms that can be postulated to explain the effects of otitis media on language. Third, we will describe some of the results on language of a few of the pertinent variables of host and pathogen at different times in a person's life span. This will be followed by a consideration of some of the data that reflects the persistence of the effect of otitis media on language, and then a concluding summary.

HISTORY

It has long been known that hearing loss during the first few years of life will result in abnormal oral language. People with less than severe to profound hearing loss will usually not be exposed to or adopt non-auditory verbal languages so that their overall linguistic abilities are diminished. Bond (1935), in a doctoral thesis, found that first and second grade New York City school children who had minor hearing losses, assumed to be associated with otitis media (OM), were poorer readers and were retained in grade more than those with normal hearing. Of interest was that among the poor readers, there were two groups, those who were initially taught with auditory instruction and those who were taught with a visually based method. Hearing loss was found only in the poor readers who were taught with the auditory method and not in the children taught with the visual system. These observations, suggesting that a hearing loss would result in poor reading and the awareness of the other deleterious effect of hearing loss led to hearing testing in schools.

The specific association of OM with language development appears to have been first articulated and documented by Vanja Holm, M.D. and LuVern Kunze, Ph.D. (1969) in their landmark paper on the effect of chronic otitis media on language and speech development. They studied two matched populations (16 children in each group) of 5- to 9-year olds of a low socio-economic class. One group had documented otitis media and associated hearing loss and the other was free of ear disease and hearing loss. They found that the children with otitis media and a history of (including some persistent) hearing loss had significant language delay in 8/8 measures of language, although there was no delay in 4/4 measures of visual and motor skills. This article reported on children who, by and large, had their hearing loss for most of their lives, an aspect of the Holm and Kunze communication that has not often been appreciated in the several hundred articles that have come out either in developing their concept or reacting to it. There has been, on the surface, a substantial contrariety of observations since the 1969 paper. Sometimes differences have been reported from the same center and the same population, depending on the age of the child and the characteristics that were measured.

MECHANISMS

There are a number of ways in which OM could have a negative impact on language. The most likely factor is the hearing loss, which fluctuates, varying as to the amount, the spectrum—that is, the frequency—and the time course. This fluctuating hearing loss occurs in infants whose speech discrimination requires a greater signal-to-noise ratio than the older child's or adult's (Nozza, Rossman, and Bond 1991; Nozza and Henson 1999; Nozza 1995). Infants require a much louder signal to equal the speech discrimination of an adult. An adult has 80% discrimination at about 7 dB hearing loss (HL), and an infant does not achieve that level of discrimination until the HL is 50dB. If there is a 20 dB attenuation, such as seen regularly in OM or otitis media with effusion (OME), the infant is able to discriminate between phonemes /ba/ versus /da/ about 60% of the time, or 10% greater than chance (Gravel and Nozza 1997). The hearing loss from OM or OME greatly diminishes the ability of a child to recognize speech as measured by the "articulation index" (AI). In this study, speech intelligibility was reduced to 0.32 with a pure tone average (PTA) loss of 40 dB (Gravel and Nozza 1997)—a small (20 dB) hearing loss creates greater difficulty in speech discrimination for the infant than for the older child or adult. To the degree that auditory deprivation can degrade oral language, infants and young children with the fluctuating hearing loss from OME will be so affected. Modest hearing losses are associated with reduction in babbling, production of simpler syllable structure, limited production of multisyllabic structures, and a limited phonetic repertoire (Schwartz, Mody, and Petinou 1997).

Observations, detailed later, show that the earliest observed language deficiencies associated with OME are delays in expressive language. This is a paradox—why should the hearing loss of OME lead to problems in expression and not perception or comprehension? It will be seen that some of the traces—an OME palimpsest—will be found in perception at age 9 years, but that does not totally answer the riddle. A plausible answer is that the limitation of babbling associated with the hearing loss will result in an impoverishment of early word complexity and vocabulary.

There are other suggested models. Shriberg and Smith (1983) suggest two other mechanisms. In the first, called the *downstream effect*, there is an unstable perception of a phoneme such as /h/ because of fluctuating hearing loss, and it is hypothesized that this perceptual deficit will lead to difficulty in learning the pronouns he, him, her, etc. Shriberg and Smith's second mechanism is termed the *indirect* or *mediated pathway*. This postulates that difficulty in hearing a signal will cause the child to pay more attention to deciphering the degraded signal and thus reduce the capacity for deeper language processing.

Two other concepts have been offered by Vernon-Feagans (1999), which take into account both the infant hearing data and other extrinsic and intrinsic factors associated with language development. The first is a hypothesis of the Global Language Model: the mild to moderate hearing loss of OME causes a periodic degradation of language input, initially causing poorer language and speech discrimination ability. The long-term consequences of the degraded or perverted discrimination are poorer verbal skills. Her second paradigm, Interactive Language and Attention Model, incorporates the Global Language Model, and is more complex in its integration of a number of variables into the model. In taking into account both intrinsic and extrinsic elements that coordinate to create the language configuration of the child, The Interactive Language and Attention model may more accurately account for the data, conceptualized as it is upon the interaction between host and pathogen.

HOST AND PATHOGEN

Almost all children have OM, but not all appear to have a resultant language deviance. To understand why some are negatively affected linguistically and others are not, it may useful to consider that disease occurs—is apparent—when the virulence of the pathogen exceeds the resistance of the host. The strength of both pathogen and the host are determined by extrinsic and intrinsic characteristics. Otitis media's role in relation to language is that of a pathogen. The resultant language outcome can be understood in the terms of host and pathogen, intrinsic and extrinsic characteristics, and interactions. This form of analysis may help to explain why some are sick—have a language deficiency—and others are not.

Children, the hosts to the pathogen OM, vary in their susceptibility by their exposure to positive and negative extrinsic factors, such as whether they have been breast-fed, been in day care, lived in a household with a smoker, etc. Increased intrinsic susceptibility for OM may derive from certain craniofacial abnormalities, immune deficiencies, and/or perhaps most commonly, a genetic predisposition to OM. The Casselbrant et al. (1999) study of twins and triplets shows a high correlation for hereditability of OME and acute otitis media for the monozygotes when compared to the dizygotes. The hearing loss, probably the most important aspect of the pathogen, varies with regard to its magnitude and amount of time in which the child is exposed to diminished hearing (Roberts et al. 1995a).

Hearing loss associated with OM in children who have other intrinsic cognitive deficiencies appears to have a greater effect on communications skills than in the normal child. There is data that shows that negative factors in the extrinsic linguistic and social environment will exacerbate the effect of OM on various language related skills. Some of the data from three studies will demonstrate this phenomenon. Shriberg et al. (2000a; 2000b) used the same metrics, a critical control, to evaluate the effect of OM on a population of Midwestern middle class pediatric clinic children and a Native American population living on a reservation. The middle class children appeared to have no linguistic consequence from the OM, whereas the Native American children showed a 4.63 increased of odds ratio for language deficiency in children with OM. The greatest difference between the groups was that the middle class children were ". . . in a language rich environment . . ."whereas the Native Americans were in " environments which may not mitigate the effects chronic discomfort or hearing loss of OME." Roberts et al. (1995b; 2000) have shown that in a population of lower socio-economic status (SES) African American children, in a special day care setting, the language skills of one-year olds were negatively correlated with their hearing loss but positively correlated with their mothers' IQ. These same children, some years later, were assessed for a language skill—recognizing incomplete words. The greater the time with hearing loss during the first years of life, the poorer the children performed on this language task. There was, however, a positive correlation with the quality of the home environment; home environments that provided richer linguistic stimulation were correlated with the children's success in recognizing incomplete words. The third study (Wallace et al. 1996) looked at four measures of expressive language in two-year olds. These children, all with documented otitis media and hearing history during their first year of life, and with study of parental language practices, were divided into four groups. All were children from low SES who had normal hearing and were free of OM after their first year. Their expressive language skills were tested at two years of age. The children with high prevalence of OM (OM+) during their first year had significant expressive language deficiency only when they also had a mother with poor communications skills. The children who were free of OM (OM–) during their first year had good expressive language regardless of their mother's communication skills. This shows that the synergy of an inadequate external sensory environment and pathogen —the OM—causes the disease—deficient expressive language at two years of age. Other studies (Brookhouser and Goldgar 1987; Freeark et al. 1992) have found a similar relation between impoverished linguistic environment and OM resulting in deficient language, whereas an adequate linguistic environment appears to ameliorate or "protect" the child from these disadvantageous sequelae.

These observations are congruent in showing that there will be a resultant language deficit when the host—the child—has OM and develops in an inadequate sensory environment; they demonstrate the interaction between biology, the OM, and culture, the child's linguistic and social milieu.

PERSISTENCE OF AN EFFECT

Adaptation and compensation are prime functions of our plastic nervous systems, especially during the period of maximum development—

early childhood. They operate both to achieve normal growth and to repair or to make up for various deficits so that the negative effect is minimized. These functions are operant in language development. In addition, as the child becomes older, the structure of his or her language changes so that the types of deficiencies found at 2 or 3 years may not be apparent in the more developed language at 8 or 9 years. There can be other manifestations and measures of language deficiencies at these older ages. Three separate research groups have reported depressed expressive language as a result of OM at 1 to 3 years of age (Shriberg et al. 2000b; Rach, Zielhuis, and van den 1988; Wallace et al. 1988). The deficiency of expressive language in the first few years appears to be one of the more constant linguistic sequelae of OM. As the child ages, this particular effect disappears (Gravel and Wallace 1992) and other defects appear. Roberts has hypothesized that the changes observed at 5 years may come about from the impairment of phonological skills, working memory, and auditory processing which now manifest as deficiencies in school readiness, verbal math, and recognition of incomplete words. Home and childcare environments diminish in their influence on language skills at age 5 years, perhaps because of the greater initial role of caretakers, and new importance of the school environment (Roberts et al. 2000).

A series of reports from the Albert Einstein College of Medicine has demonstrated the changing manifestations over a 9 year period of the OM and associated hearing loss that occurred only during the first year of life (Wallace et al. 1988; Gravel and Wallace 1992; Abraham, Wallace, and Gravel 1996; Gravel, Wallace, and Ruben 1995; Gravel and Wallace 1995; Mody et al. 1999; Ruben, Wallace, and Gravel 1997; Wallace et al. 1988; Wallace and Hooper 1997). These children, from low SES, have all been followed prospectively from birth though their 9th year, and are still being followed as adolescents. They were divided into two groups that differed only with regard to whether they had very little otitis media and hearing loss (OM–) or frequent otitis media and associated hearing loss (OM+) during their first year of life. The average ABR hearing thresholds differed 11dB between the two groups. The OM+ had normal threshold 8% of the time as compared to the OM–, who had normal threshold 38% of the time during the first year of life. For the remainder of the study—to age nine years and older—these children were free of otitis media and had normal hearing. The OM+ children were not among the most severely affected in terms of a typical clinical population, as their OM was relatively mild. At one year of age, as noted above, a delay was identified in their expressive language but not in their receptive language. At two years, the effects of the good and poor communication practices of the mothers were related to good and poor expressive language in the OM+ group.

At 4 years of age the OM+ needed 3dB greater signal-to-noise ratio to understand a sentence. The 3 dB deficit in signal-to-noise ratio can result in a 30% decrease in speech intelligibility.

At 6 years of age the children who were OM+ during their first year of life were found to be at greater academic risk than the ones who were OM–. The competitive listening tasks noted at 4 years of age were related to the academic subscale of the SIFTER test at age 6. It is inferred that these OM+ children were at a constant disadvantage in the classroom because of their deficit in signal discrimination in the context of background noise.

Tests of the two groups, OM+ and OM–, at 9 years of age showed that the OM+ children had significant difficulty in verbal memory as measured by temporal order judgment. This was consistent with the previous data, in that these children had difficulty with the perception of speech in noise and in detecting phonetically similar tasks. Klausen's (Klausen et al. 2000) data were congruent with the Einstein College of Medicine observations in their findings of significantly lower scores in an articulation test and small, but significantly lower scores in the test regarding sound discrimination. No significant differences on other language skills were detected by the ITPA test or Boston naming test. This group also found a significantly higher degree of right ear advantage and lower attentional effectiveness in the OME- group.

So far, all of the data that has been presented has been that of groups of children. The health care provider, however, is concerned with the individual. Responsibility for populations lies with the commonweal, usually effected through a governmental agency. To answer the question, "What were the effects of early OM on a child's language abilities?" the data for each of the individual Einstein children were analyzed. The goal was to determine whether there was a consistent effect throughout the nine years, or were there just a few children with large deviances that caused the statistical variance in the groups (OM– vs. OM+) (Ruben 1999). The percentage of days for which each of the OM+ children had OME was compared with that of the OM– children. These OM+ children were affected on the average six times more frequently than the OM–. Then each child's eight language assessments, measured over the course of nine years, was compared to the average of the OM– subjects. Two subjects, WE and ME, are typical of the group. Only one of the eight evaluations over the nine years of two subjects had a language assessment that was equally as good as the OM– average. When each of the OM+ children was analyzed over the nine years, it was found that a few scored, on occasion, equal to or better in language measures than the average of the OM– children during the same nine years of assessment. At age 4 it was found that a third of the OM+ children were equal to or better than the average OM– children. As they became older, however, the OM+ disadvantage appears even more clearly. The percentage of evaluations of OM+ children who fared less well on linguistic tests than the OM– children ranges from 63% to 100%. The percentage of OM+ children who fared less well than the OM– in all evaluations ranged from 75% to 100%. In sum, most of the OM+ children performed worse than the OM– children during the nine years of follow up, and most OM+ children performed consistently worse for the nine years when compared to the mean of the control group. The effect persists at least to the ninth year of life and was essentially constant in each child.

Do these measurable and persistent effects of early OM have a communication consequence that is of negative significance for the individual and society? This question has been examined in two large population studies (Bennett and Haggard 1999) that are important (Luotonen et al. 1998a) because the large populations provide the statistical power to observe small but significant differences. The Finnish study (Luotonen et al. 1998a) of 1,708 children compared those with and without OM during the first three years on nine measures at 8 and 9 years of age. It was found that the OM+ children were, with statistical significance, below the median in 5 of the nine measures: narrative writing, mechanical reading, reading comprehension, oral performance, and attention skills. These results, from a large population, are consistent with the more detailed studies carried out with smaller numbers of subjects in that these deficits can be related to problems in detecting the signal—speech—in noise. The Finnish study, in contrast to work done in the United States, was carried out in a relatively homogenous population, and did not find any correlation with maternal education, nor with birth order.

A study from the United Kingdom (Bennet and Haggard 1999) followed a birth cohort, born between the 5th and the 11th of April 1970, for 10 years. They analyzed the data of 12,000 children at 5 years, and of 9,000 children at 10 years. Two of their outcome measures were behavior and language. This comprehensive population study showed negative effects of OM on both behavior and language at 5 and 10 years of age. These differences were found to be independent of social background and other extrinsic variables. In both of these large population studies, the Finnish and the English, the effects are small, though not insignificant, within the individual, and they are shown to affect a large portion of the population. A recent report (Paradise et al. 2001) purports to show that children younger than three years of age who have persistent otitis media and received a prompt insertion of tympanostomy tubes did not measurably improve language and other developmental outcomes at the age of three years.

This prospective study excluded most, if not all, of the children who might have extrinsic or intrinsic risk host and vector factors that would contribute to a language deficit. Those excluded from the study included birth weight < 5 lbs, small for gestational age, neonatal asphyxia, other serious illness, major congenital malformations, chronic illness, multiple birth, foster care, sibling enrolled, adopted, mother dead, mother known drug or alcohol abuser, mother limited socially, mother limited intellectually, mother > 18 years old, and English not the only language spoken. Additionally only 9% of their evaluated population had bilateral continuous OME, abnormal hearing loss, and tympanostomy tube insertion within 60 days. Their negative results are possibly only applicable to healthy children in good linguistic environments with minimal ear disease. These data (Paradise 2001) do not apply to the general population or to children (hosts) who are at risk because of intrinsic and/or extrinsic risk factors. The data from the English and Finnish studies (Bennett and Haggard 1998; Luotonen et al. 1998b) indicate that OM in early childhood results in decrease in the overall linguistic capacity of society as a whole; it is, furthermore, associated with deviant behavior. The consequences of these widespread deficits, which may be small on an individual basis, but which are multiplied by a vast factor, are particularly deleterious, both for the individual and society, in the communication based economy that is today and tomorrow's reality (Ruben 2000).

SUMMARY

Otitis media can be understood as both a disease itself, and as a pathogen in affecting language development. Otitis media, very common during the first three years of life, is associated with a variable and fluctuating hearing loss during the period of early language acquisition. In some children, there will be more episodes of OM than in others, and there may be greater or lesser severity. Depending on these factors, the OM will cause a greater or lesser degree of auditory distortion and auditory deprivation. The effect of this variable pathogen on the child—the host—is synergetic with factors of the child's extrinsic and intrinsic makeup. The language outcome is a function of the complexities of host/pathogen interactions. Several schema have been developed that seek to demonstrate these relationships (Vernon-Feagans 1999; Bennett and Haggard 1999). The critical pathogen properties are: the age of occurrence; the extent of the hearing loss, both intensity and frequency; the duration of the loss; and probably the variability of the hearing. The host's response and outcome are affected by the intrinsic factors of susceptibility to OM (genetic as well as intrinsic response to environmental factors such as tobacco smoke); cognitive ability; and language capability, e.g., specific language impairment (Bishop 2001). The most commonly identified and what appears to be very potent extrinsic host factor is the child's linguistic environment. In an impoverished language context, the child with OM will have a language deficit greater than the child who is in an adequate language context, who may have none that is measurable.

The care of the individual child is the day-to-day task. On what bases should decisions be made about when to intervene with a young child in regard to language function? It is reasonable to measure the language function of the child and if it is found to be deficient then an intervention can be considered. What is essential for all interventions, however, is that the outcome be measured. Did the intervention for OME result in improved language? This can be assessed with the use of a language screen before and after the intervention has been carried out (Ruben 1991).

And, going beyond the concern for the individual, the high prevalence of OM and the effects found in population studies make the linguistic deficiencies from OM a major societal issue. An effective, competitive society ensures the optimal function of its members. Who will win the economic and social races in our current communication-based culture? Those with optimal language skills. The relationship between OM and language is multifactorial, and early OM results in language deficiency, particularly for those who have prolonged hearing loss and/or are in a linguistically impoverished environment.

REFERENCES

Abraham, S. S., Wallace, I. F., and Gravel, J. S. 1996. Early otitis media and phonological development at age 2 years. *Laryngoscope* 106(6):727–32.
Bennett, K. E., and Haggard, M. P. 1998. Accumulation of factors influencing children's middle ear disease: Risk factor modeling on a large population cohort. *Journal of Epidemiology and Community Health* 52:786–93.
Bennett, K. E., and Haggard, M. P. 1999. *Archives of the Disabled Child* 80(1):28–35.
Bishop, D. V. M. 2001. Genetic and environmental risks for specific language impairment in children. *Phil Transcripts of the Royal Society of London* B356(1407):369–80.
Bond, G. L. *The Auditory and Speech Characteristics of Poor Readers.* New York: Bureau of Publication, Teachers College, Columbia University.
Brookhouser, P. E., and Goldgar, D. E. Medical profile of the language-delayed child: Otitis prone versus otitis-free. *International Journal of Pediatric Otohinolaryngology* 12(3):237–71.
Casselbrant, M. L., Mandel, E. M., Fall, P. A., Rockette, H. E., Kurs-Lasky, M., Bluestone, C. D. et al. 1999. The heritability of otitis media: A twin and triplet study. *JAMA* 282(22):2125–30.

Freeark, K., Frank, S. J., Wagner, A. E., Lopez, M., Olmstead, C., and Girard R. 1992. Otitis media, language development, and parental verbal stimulation. *Journal of Pediatric Psychology.* 17(2):173–85.

Gravel, J. S., and Nozza, R. J. 1997. Hearing loss among children with otitis media with effusion. In *Otitis Media in Young Children: Medical, Developmental and Educational Considerations,* eds. J. E. Robert, I. F. Wallace, and D. Henderson. Baltimore: Paul H Brookes.

Gravel, J. S., and Wallace, I. F. 1998. Language, speech, and educational outcomes of otitis media. *Journal of Otolaryngology* 27 Suppl 2:17–25.

Gravel, J. S., and Wallace, I. F. 1992. Listening and language at 4 years of age: Effects of early otitis media. *Journal of Speech and Hearing Research* 35(3): 588–95.

Gravel, J. S., Wallace, I. F., and Ruben, R. J. 1995. Early otitis media and later educational risk. *Acta Otolaryngology* (Stockholm) 115 (2):279–81.

Holm, V. A., and Kunze, L. H. 1969. Effect of chronic otitis media on language and speech development. *Pediatrics* 43(5):833–39.

Klausen, O., Moller, P., Holmefjord, A., Reisaeter, S., and Asbjornsen, A. 2000. *Acta Otolaryngology* 73–76.

Luotonen, M., Uhari, M., Aitola, L., Lukkaroinen, A. M., Luotonen, J., and Uhari, M. 1998. A nation-wise, population-based survey of otitis media and school achievement. *International Journal of Pediatric Otohinolaryngology* 43(1):41–51.

Mody, M., Schwartz, R. G., Gravel, J. S., and Ruben, R. J. 1999. Speech perception and verbal memory in children with and without histories of otitis media. *Journal of Speech, Language, & Hearing Research* 42(5):1069–79.

Nozza, R. J. 1995. Estimating the contribution of non-sensory factors to infant-adult differences in behavioral thresholds. *Hearing Research* 91(1–2):72–78.

Nozza, R. J., and Henson, A. M. 1999. Unmasked thresholds and minimum masking in infants and adults: Separating sensory from nonsensory contributions to infant-adult differences in behavioral thresholds. *Ear and Hearing* 20(6):483–96.

Nozza, R. J., Rossman, R. N., and Bond, L. C. 1991. Infant-adult differences in unmasked thresholds for the discrimination of consonant-vowel syllable pairs. *Audiology* 30(2):102–12.

Paradise, J. L., Feldman, H. M., Campbell, T. F., Dollaghan, C. A., Colborn, D. K., Bernard, B. S., et al. 2001. Effect of early and delayed insertion of tympanostomy tubes for persistent otitis media on developmental outcomes at the age of three years. *New England Journal of Medicine* 344(16) 1179–87.

Rach, G. H., Zielhuis, G. A., and van den, B. P. 1988. The influence of chronic persistent otitis media with effusion on language development of 2- to 4-year -olds. *International Journal of Pediatric Otorhinolaryngology* 15(3):253–61.

Roberts, J. E., Burchinal, M. R., Medley, L. P., Zeisen, S. A., Mundy, M., Roush, J., et al. 1995. Otitis media, hearing sensitivity, and maternal responsiveness in relation to language during infancy. *Journal of Pediatrics* 126(3): 481–89.

Roberts, J. E., Burchinal, M. R., Jackson, S. C., Hooper, S. R., Roush, J., Mundy, M., et al. 2000. Otitis media in early childhood in relation to preschool language and school readiness skills among black children. *Pediatrics* 106(4): 725–35.

Ruben, R. J. 1991. Language screening as a factor in the management of the pediatric otolaryngic patient: Effectiveness and efficiency. *Archives of Otolaryngology Head and Neck Surgery* 117(9):1021–25.

Ruben, R. J. 1999. Persistency of an effect: Otitis media during the first year of life with nine years follow-up. *International Journal of Otorhinolaryngology* 49 Suppl 1:S115–S118.

Ruben, R. J., Wallace, I. F., and Gravel, J. 1997. Long-term communication deficiencies in children with otitis media during their first year of life. *Acta Otolaryngology* (Stockholm) 117(2):206–07.

Ruben, R. J. 2000. Redefining the survival of the fittest: Communication disorders in the 21st century. *Laryngoscope* 110(2Pt 1):241–45.

Schwartz, R., Mody, M., and Petinou, K. 1997. Phonological acquisition and otitis media. In *Otitis Media in Young Children*, eds. J. Roberts, I. F. Wallace, and F. W. Henderson. Baltimore: Paul H. Brookes.

Shriberg, L. D., and Smith, A. J. 1983. Phonological correlates of middle-ear involvement in speech-delayed children: A methodological note. *Journal of Speech and Hearing Research* 26(2):293–97.

Shriberg, L. D., Friel-Patti, S., Flipsen, J., Jr., and Brown, R. L. 2000. Otitis media, fluctuant hearing loss, and speech-language outcomes, A preliminary structural equation model. *Journal of Speech, Language & Hearing Research* 43:100–120.

Shriberg, L. D., Flipsen, P., Jr., Thielke, H., Kwiatkowski, J., Kertoy, M. K., Katcher, M. L. et al. 2000. Risk for speech disorder associated with early recurrent otitis media with effusion: Two retrospective studies. *Journal of Speech, Language & Hearing Research* 43(1):79–99.

Vernon-Feagans, L. 1999. Impact of otitis media on speech, language, cognition, and behavior. In *Evidence-based Otitis Media*, eds. R. M. Rosenfeld and C. D. Bluestone Hamilton: B. C. Decker.

Wallace, I. F., and Hooper, S. R. 1997. Otitis media and its impact on cognitive, academic, and behavioral outcomes, A review and interpretation of the findings. In *Otitis Media in Young Children*, eds. J. E. Roberts, I. F. Wallace, and F. W. Henderson. Baltimore: Paul H. Brookes Publishing Co.

Wallace, I. F., Gravel, J. S., McCarton, C. M., and Ruben, R. J. 1988. Otitis media and language development at 1 year of age. *International Journal of Pediatric Otorhinolaryngology* 15(3):253–61.

Wallace, I. F., Gravel, J. S., Schwartz, R. G., and Ruben, R. J. 1996. Otitis media, communication style of primary caregivers, and language skill of 2 year olds: A preliminary report. *Journal of Developmental and Behavioral Pediatrics* 17(1):27–35.

Wallace, I. F., Gravel, J. S., McCarton, C. M., Stapells, D. R., Bernstein, R. S., and Ruben, R. J. 1988. Otitis media, auditory sensitivity, and language outcomes of one year. *Laryngoscope* 98(1):64–70.

Part • III

Medical Diagnosis

Chapter • 6

A Neurodevelopmental Approach to the Child with Delayed Language

Mary L. O'Connor Leppert

The acquisition of language is a complex, multifaceted process that commences at birth (or earlier), and in the normal course of development evolves into a sophisticated cognitive process that is the essence of human interaction. If language does not develop normally, the child is placed at a great disadvantage in the world that surrounds him. The impact of delayed or abnormal language development on the child and his caregivers varies in degree, presentation, and effect, and therefore is worthy of thorough evaluation.

NORMAL LANGUAGE DEVELOPMENT

Development of normal language starts with the establishment of a word lexicon or repository of words that begins to be formed at birth. Newborns naïve to verbal stimuli are gradually exposed to a vocabulary that expands with advancing age. The earliest exposure to vocabulary is a limited repertoire of words used at a close physical range and spoken with a soft tone. A warm parental facial expression is the visual stimulus that accompanies the words. The same limited vocabulary is repeated to the infant in his or her parent's arms for the first few months of life. As the infant's world expands with increasing motor ability and visual ability, he or she is exposed to a broader range of vocabulary including objects, people, toys, and pets that are labeled repeatedly by the parents. Tone changes from one full of emotion to declarative labeling. As motor skills expand, exposure to the number of labeled objects increases, and the lexicon expands. By the time a child begins to crawl, not only has the vocabulary expanded, but so too have the tones used to convey information. The tone associated with "NO!" is a novel one and provides a new inference to a single word that is sufficient for stopping the toddler from creeping up the stairs or touching an electrical outlet. Credit for acquisition of the first spoken word is given to the child when he or she utters his or her first word at about 11 or 12 months of age. Though the beginning of a demonstrable vocabulary is present at about a year, most of the single word utterances used in the next few months will, in effect, be labeling of visual stimuli. A child will say "dog" when a dog enters the visual field, but will not say "dog" spontaneously because he or she desires to see the dog. Spontaneous use of single words, and the early efforts of combining two words to a phrase, demonstrate not only the establishment of a word repository, but also the ability to summon language without a visual stimulus. Parents continue to label for children throughout the toddler and preschool years, as the child's use of language becomes more sophisticated and independent.

The late Mary Sheridan described the prerequisites for the establishment of a word repository and language development: At a most basic physiologic level, adequate hearing is vital for the reception of verbally presented information. The second requirement is the ability to listen. Listening is dependent on adequate hearing, appropriate attention, and the capacity to direct attention to foreground verbal information while ignoring background noise or conversation. The third requirement for language is sufficient intellect to absorb new information, to retrieve pre-existing verbal information, and to interpret it correctly. As the ultimate goal of language development is communication, it follows that the final requirement for normal language development is the desire to establish rapport with others (Sheridan 1964).

Higher-level language abilities required for the analysis of syntax, pragmatics, and semantics, when compromised, can be impairing on a different level than the more common disorders of expressive and receptive language. Children with higher language disorders may develop normally the expressive and receptive skills for adequate verbal communication, but may lack understanding of information that is not presented at a literal or concrete level. Failure to appreciate tone of voice, prosody of speech, body language, or the inferences made by sarcasm or humor leaves a child understanding only the most literal form of communication. These disorders of higher language may be associated with impaired basic language development and may be observed in the preschool years, or may occur with relatively little compromise of the establishment of the lexicon and expressive use of language; in this case, the higher language disorder goes undetected until the demands of abstract language or inferential thinking increase.

MEASUREMENT OF LANGUAGE DEVELOPMENT

In all streams of development the use of milestone attainment is the mainstay of a developmental assessment. Development of language is measured by sequential levels of understanding and use of vocabulary. Expressive language development has three stages: guttural, prelinguistic, and linguistic (Capute 1996). In the first or guttural stage all the vocalizations of the infant are physiologic. A child may sneeze, cry, burp, and sigh, but none of these vocalizations is an attempt at socializing. The guttural stage gives way to the prelinguistic stage with the social smile, which is an effort by the infant to respond to his parents' communication. The social smile is the first evidence that the infant recognizes interaction with others. Cooing, ah-gooing, razzing, laughing, and babbling follow the social smile as vocalized attempts to communicate, before the use of any established vocabulary. The linguistic phase of expressive language development commences with the first word use at about 11 or 12 months of age. The use of the first word occurs simultaneously with the specific use of Mama and Dada. In the next 6 months of life there is slow acquisition of single word use; by about 21 months the child begins to use phrases. Vocabulary then grows exponentially—words are connected in sentences and the child is launched to a new level of communication.

The appreciation of language understanding, or receptive language, may be demonstrated by milestones as well. From birth, the infant is alert to sounds (ringing a bell). Eyes widen, there is a momentary interruption of the movement or a change in physiologic measures (pulse, respirations) that show awareness of the sound. By four months, an infant turns to mother's voice, shortly after this, will turn the head (lateralize) to the source of the bell, but not localize the bell. By seven months, the source of the bells ring is localized in an indirect way (first lateralize, then localize), and finally, by nine months, the infant turns immediately to the bell in a direct way.

The first indication of language understanding is the understanding of the word "No" at 10 months. By 12 months, an infant can understand simple commands with gestures ("give me the shoes"). At 15 months, a gesture is not required to understand commands, and by 24 months, the child demonstrates understanding by following two-step commands, and by pointing to body parts and pictures.

LANGUAGE DISORDER DEFINITIONS

For the purpose of clarity of this text, some of the terms used in the description of the language-impaired child must be defined. A developmental language disorder is a primary disorder manifested by delayed acquisition of language that occurs in the absence of an attributable cause, such as limited cognition, hearing impairment, seizure disorder, motor dysfunction, and autistic spectrum disorders. The subtypes of developmental language disorder take three forms: expressive language disorder, mixed receptive and expressive language disorder, and pragmatic language disorder. A secondary language disorder is the delayed acquisition of language milestones that is explained by or attributed to an identifiable etiology. (See table I.)

Expressive language disorder is characterized by a failure to develop verbal abilities expected for a child's mental age, demonstrated by either a limited vocabulary (too few spoken words) or poor quality of speech. Speech disorders include phonological, articulation, voice, or fluency difficulties, or, in its most severe form, verbal dyspraxia. Essential to the diagnosis of expressive language disorder is the presence of normal comprehension of language.

Mixed receptive and expressive language disorder is a failure to comprehend verbally presented information at a level expected for a child's cognitive ability. It is logical that a child who has a poor or compromised understanding of language will have difficulty with its expression. Some expressive difficulties are always present with receptive language delay, and with rare exception, receptive language abilities exceed expressive abilities. Children with receptive language disorder may therefore present with a chief complaint of not speaking at an age appropriate level, or as a perceived difficulty with hearing, listening, following commands, or interpreting commands. Some children are seen as disobedient, because of noncompliance with following direction, or as inattentive, because they do not appear to be listening, when in fact, they listen but simply do not understand the verbally presented information.

Pragmatic language disorders seen in young children, unlike higher order language dysfunction in an older child, is generally accompanied by difficulty with receptive and expressive skills. In the

Table I.   Types of Language Disorders

Primary Language Disorders

- Expressive- Language- vocabulary
                 Speech - Phonation
                            Articulation
                            Fluency
                            Voicing
- Mixed Receptive and Expressive
- Pragmatic

Secondary Language Disorders

most severe form, pragmatic language disorder in the toddler is part of the autistic spectrum complex of symptoms. Language in this instance may appear pedantic, perseverative, or lack reciprocity. The child may not appreciate tone that conveys emotion and this may add to the frustration of the caregivers.

LANGUAGE DELAY: THE PRESENTING COMPLAINT

Independent of the etiology or type of language delay, most children with language delay see their pediatrician because of their parent's concern that, "Billy doesn't talk like other children his age." By the time a parent brings a child to the attention of the medical profession with complaints of language delay, verification of the complaint is unnecessary, and screening evaluations are redundant. The backyard screening of children by their parents (comparing Billy to every sibling, niece, nephew, and playmate) has been completed, and the parent's estimation of their child's developmental level is remarkably accurate (Pulsifer et al. 1994).

The etiology of language delay should be the primary focus of the pediatrician, as identification of an attributable cause is vital to the prognosis and management of the problem. The age at which a child with delayed language is seen by a clinician does not give any clues as to the etiology of the delay. The three main causes of language delay—mental retardation, hearing impairment, and primary developmental language disorders—present with the same chief complaint at approximately the same age. Language delay secondary to impaired cognition shows up at an average age of 27 months; primary language delay, at an average age of 32 months (Lock et al. 1986).

HISTORY

As is the case in most disorders that are seen by pediatricians for medical assessment, the clues to diagnosis often are discovered in the information gathered while taking a careful history. In a child with the chief complaint of delayed language, the goal of the history is to establish historical risk for language delay (which may point to diagnosis) and to look for historical evidence of delay in expression and understanding of language, as well as delays in the other streams of development.

Assessment of risk is sought in the birth history by inquiring about infections, toxins, prematurity, hyperbilirubinaemia, and other prenatal and perinatal complications. Past medical history would seek risk for language delay in the face of serious infection, trauma, seizure disorder, and chronic medical conditions. Family history of late talk-ers, mental retardation, hearing impairments, genetic syndromes, learning disabilities, and autism can be strongly associated with chil-dren delayed in language. Finally, though fortunately rarely, social/ environmental deprivation may play a role in the delayed acquisition of language.

A developmental history must include a review of all aspects of development: gross motor, visual motor, language, social skills, and adaptive skills. A physician must always consider that the presenting complaint may be the "tip of the iceberg," highlighting only one com-ponent of a more generalized disorder of development. Language delay is an obvious symptom of mental retardation, where all streams of development, with the possible exception of motor development, are delayed. Language delay can also be a co-morbid symptom in the disorders of cerebral palsy, autism, pervasive developmental disorder (PDD), and other developmental disorders, so to serve the child prop-erly, the whole picture of development must be brought into focus. Disordered language may be the foundation of behavioral disorders as well. A final point about the developmental history is the impor-tance of inquiring about loss of skills. The presence of a history of loss of milestones changes the tone of the evaluation, focuses the medical work up, and expands the differential diagnosis and prognosis.

Inquiry must also be made into the presence of problems fre-quently associated with language delay, and disorders of which lan-guage delay is a component. The presence of associated behavioral and mood problems may help determine the presence of co-morbid conditions such as attention deficit/hyperactivity disorder (ADHD), oppositional defiant disorder (ODD), obsessive-compulsive disorder (OCD), and affective disorders. The history of concurrent behavioral problems, stereotypies, or social or adaptive deficits may indicate that the language delay is part of a broader spectrum disorder such as mental retardation, autism, or pervasive developmental disorder.

PHYSICAL EXAMINATION

The value of a physical examination in a language-delayed child is fre-quently limited, but should be a routine part of every evaluation to rule out medical conditions that are associated with language disor-der. The general physical examination should include a review of growth parameters (including head circumference), dysmorphic fea-tures, craniofacial structures, and neurocutaneous markers. Specific syndromes the pediatrician should consider in reviewing dysmorphic features in the language-delayed child include fragile X syndrome, veliocardiofacial syndrome, Opitz syndromes and many of the mental retardation syndromes. Dysmorphisms associated with fetal exposure to alcohol and other toxins should be noted and verified with the history of pregnancy. A neurodevelopmental examination requires review of cranial nerves, tone, deep tendon reflexes, primitive, and postural reactions in the infant, and soft signs in the older child. Though it is unusual to elicit hard neurologic signs in language-delayed children, soft neurological signs are very frequent findings.

Critical assessment of the historical information and physical examination is the first step to sift out identifiable causes of language delay from primary language delay. All children reviewed for delayed understanding require a hearing evaluation, whether concern regarding adequate hearing is present or absent. The physical examination and history should eliminate clear attributable causes of language delay such as motor impairment, clinically apparent syndrome complexes, seizure disorders, environmental deprivation, and autistic spectrum disorders. Medical investigations should include a thorough evaluation of hearing in all children with language delay. Further medical assessment looking for etiology is dictated by history and physical examination. Probes for fragile X syndrome, veliocardiofacial syndrome, or general karyotyping may be suggested because of noted dysmorphisms or because of associated physical findings such as cardiac defects or palatal defects. An EEG may be appropriate in the presence of staring spells, overt seizure, or language loss. Metabolic testing is indicated with loss of skills, coarse features, or visceromegaly. An important cause of language delay that may not be clarified by history and physical examination or by further medical testing is mental retardation. Mental retardation can only be differentiated from developmental language disorder by assessment of visual motor and adaptive skills during the neurodevelopmental assessment.

NEURODEVELOPMENTAL ASSESSMENT

"In the normal infant development is methodical, orderly and timed; it goes through a gradient that can be divided into orderly sequences which can follow each other with such regularity that they are in the main predictable" (Gesell and Amatruda 1947).

Neurodevelopmental testing includes both quantitative and qualitative measures. The aspects of development that should be quantified include the cognitive streams of language and visual motor skills, as well as adaptive, social, and gross motor scales. Each aspect of development must be assessed individually, then reviewed to assess overall development. When children develop abnormally, they do so in one or more of three patterns: delay, deviancy, and dissociation. In developmental delay, the normal sequence of milestone achievement is seen, but the rate of achievement is slower than normal. Delay may occur in a single stream of development or across several or all streams. Deviancy is an abnormal sequence of milestone attainment within a given stream. An example in motor development would be a child who crawls (8 month skill) before he sits (6 month skill). Deviancy in a given stream is not of diagnostic value, but alerts the examiner to the presence of an underlying disorder. Finally, dissociation is a phenomenon of differing rates of development across the five streams of development. A child with cerebral palsy may have normal rates of development in cognition, adaptive skills, and social skills, but a delayed (and therefore dissociated) rate in gross motor development. (See table II.)

Qualitative assessments are made during clinical observations of a child's language, behavior, and activity, and are noted in the child's history and physical, and neurodevelopmental testing. Assessment of expressive language use—phonation, intonation, articulation, vocabulary depth, echolalia, fluency, and verbal perseveration—takes place during interaction with the child in the pediatric assessment. A sense of receptive language skills will also be made apparent by the child's ability to follow commands, follow conversation directed at his or her level, and reciprocate in conversation that is relevant. Behavioral observations of eye contact, attention, activity level, and play skills are difficult to quantify, but add very important subjective information. Likewise, pragmatic deficits (appreciation of tone of voice, body language, respect for others' space, etc.) may be subtle, but obvious to the alert observer. All these observations, taken in context of history and quantitative assessment, give the clinician additional premises for a diagnosis, and permit inferences about associated conditions.

TEST MEASURES

Test measures employed for quantifying development must assess both of the cognitive streams—language and visual motor skills—in order to differentiate language delay as a primary diagnosis from a secondary phenomenon of a more global intellectual deficiency. Many tests are appropriate for assessment, so choice may be made based on

Table II. Developmental Principles

Delay
Deviancy
Dissociation

the preferences and training of the assessor, the time available for testing, and the information sought in testing. Cognition evaluation absolutely requires that verbal and nonverbal or visual motor skills be measured separately and that each stream be quantified. If previous cognitive testing is available and valid, then assessment may be limited to language skills. In this case, the test(s) employed should measure both expressive and receptive skills. Measurements of associated behavioral, adaptive, and social abilities may be required and are usually ascertained in the form of checklists or rating scales.

A widely accepted standard for measurement of cognition in infants and toddlers is the Bayley Scales of Infant Development II (BSID II) (Bayley 1969). The BSID II measures language and visual motor skills independently, and gives an overall score called the Mental Development Index (MDI). The BSID II, though optimal for assessment, is impractical for use in the primary care setting, as it requires a generous amount of time and a trained psychologist to administer it. The Stanford Binet IV (SB-IV) (Stanford Binet), like the BSID II, is a good cognitive measure, but is also time consuming and is generally administered by a psychologist. Developmental scales available for use by the primary care physician that also measure language and visual motor skills include the Denver Developmental Screening Test II (DDST-II) (Frankenburg et al. 1992) and the Capute Scales or the CAT/CLAMS, among others. A wide variety of tools for the assessment of language in the infant and toddler may be employed in the primary care office; among these are the Early Language Milestone Scale (ELMS) (Coplan 1993), and the Peabody Picture Vocabulary Test (PPVT).

THE CAPUTE SCALES

Arnold Capute derived the Capute Scales, known formerly as the Cognitive Adaptive Test/Clinical Linguistic and Auditory Milestone Scale (CAT/CLAMS) from milestones on tests initially designed by Arnold Gesell. Gesell's test of development (Knobloch and Pasamanick 1974) in 1929 was extensive, consisting of 195 test items in the first 30 months of life. Gesell's work endured many revisions by such researchers as Cattell (Catell 1940), Illingsworth (Illingsworth 1987), Sheridan (Sheridan 1968), and Bayley (Bayley 1993). The Bayley Scales of Infant Development (BSID) of 1969 was revised in 1993 to the BSID II, which remains a current standard for infant and toddler assessment.

The Capute Scales were initially evaluated in a normative population and were shown to have significant correlation with the Bayley Mental Development Index (MDI) on 24 of the 25 milestones tested (Capute, Palmer, Shapiro et al. 1986). The Capute Scales have shown to have concurrent and predictive validity in a number of studies in high-risk populations when compared with standard measures of cognition (Capute, Shapiro, Wachtel et al. 1986; Hoon et al. 1993; Wachtel, Shapiro, Palmer et al. 1994; Wachtel, Topper, Houck et al. 1994; Kube et al. 2000). More recent studies on the Capute Scales have been aimed at populations of children not known to have risk for developmental disorders. These studies also indicate that the Capute scales are an effective instrument for the identification of toddlers with developmental delay, and compare favorably to standardized measures (Leppert et al. 1998). Presently, the Capute Scales are being standardized again in a large normative population to strengthen their basis for use in the general pediatrics office (Accardo 2002).

The language section of the Capute scales, the CLAMS, is a measurement of both receptive and expressive language milestones in the first three years of life. The CLAMS scale has four important benefits that make it extremely useful in primary care assessments: receptive and expressive skills are taken from parental history for the first 18 months of life; a paucity of instruments are needed (blocks and a picture card); delay can be quantified using a developmental quotient; and deviancy in receptive and expressive steams can be elicited. The advantage of taking language skill measurement from parental history is obvious to anyone practiced in the art of trying to cajole even the most talkative child to speak in the office setting. The cost of this convenience to the practitioner is that the language history must be taken meticulously to ensure its accuracy. There are several specific milestones that may overestimate the child's language abilities, and these should be evaluated carefully. In the mid-prelinguistic stage children develop babbling, although in the later prelinguistic stage, mama and dada are spoken non-specifically, then specifically in the early linguistic stage. Care must be taken to differentiate the use of "dada" as it can be part of a babbling string, "da-da-da-da," or a non-specific label "dada," or a specific label "Dada" used for the child's father. Similarly in the second and third years of life we ask parents to estimate the extent of their child's vocabulary. Clarity is required to ascertain the size of the vocabulary as proper nouns or names are not included in vocabulary on the Capute language scale. History of two word phrases and two word sentences should be looked at carefully. Children should not be credited for two-word phrases when there is a single word concept. "Thank you," "hot dog," and "ice cream" are one-word concepts. Similarly, phrases must be differentiated from sentences by the use of verbs. Concurrent with the development of a vocabulary sufficient to use two-word phrases is the development of echolalia. Echolalia is a normal phenomenon in which a child will repeat the whole or a part of words he has just heard. This phenomenon begins at about 18 months of life, peaks at 24 months, and is to be considered pathological after about 30 months of life. One must be careful when asking the size of vocabulary that only spontaneously used words are counted. Words echoed are not necessarily committed to the word lexicon and children should not be credited for their use.

Accuracy in obtaining receptive language history is somewhat easier, as most receptive skills are demonstrated in the examination. Reluctance to speak in the exam setting does not seem to carry over to following commands. Children turn to the bell in a manner appropriate for their mental age when the bell sounds above and behind their ears. Generally by the time a child is able to identify body parts they do so willfully, if not for the examiner, for their parent. The receptive language skills questions that should be asked specifically deal with the child's ability to follow directions. A gesture is required at 12 months of age, but not at 15 months when a child is asked to follow a single command. Examples should be requested for how a child follows a two-step command at 24 months. The commands should be unrelated to show that the child is capable of correctly interpreting two separate bits of verbal information. "Pick up your shoes, and go shut the door" is an unrelated two-step command, while "Take your trash and put it in the bin" are related commands and follow naturally, thus, both commands are successful if the child follows the single command, "Put it in the bin."

Specific history taking is prudent to ensure accuracy of measuring language ability. However, if expressive language milestones are paired and correlate, the examiner is reassured of the accuracy of his measure. Immature jargoning (lengthy, nonsensical verbalizations that convey tone and emotion) occurs with a vocabulary of 2 to 3 words, mature jargoning (similar to immature jargoning, with a real word put into the verbalization) occurs when the vocabulary has reached about 10 words, two-word phrases develop with about 20-word vocabulary, and two-word sentences with an estimated 50 words. When these expressive milestones do not correlate, a careful review to clarify inconsistencies is suggested.

The visual motor or problem solving scale of the Capute Scales, previously referred to as the CAT scale, provides an assessment of the non-verbal cognitive abilities of children with mental ages of less than 36 months. Like the language scale, the visual motor test uses a limited number of test instruments, and each can be used over a wide range of ages. The use of a single test instrument over a large range of ages allows the examiner to start at an age level below the child's estimated function and push testing to the limit of his abilities without breaking up the examination too frequently. Cubes are employed in testing from 6 months to 36 months, the crayon from 12 months to 36 months, the form board from 16 months to 30 months, and all serve to have smooth transition through test sets in the shortest possible time. Unlike the language scale, every item on the visual motor scale must be demonstrated in the evaluation. To ensure the greatest cooperation from the child, it is advisable to begin testing several month sets below the child's estimated age of function. Beginning below a child's ability adds a small bit of time to the exam, but establishes a level of confidence in the child that encourages his attempt at higher level items. Allowing the child to have success early in the evaluation also ensures the establishment of a basal level of ability. Occasionally, it is necessary to use a parent as a proxy for the examiner to optimize co-operation of the child.

Scoring of the Capute Scales is accomplished by first establishing a basal level of ability, then adding a numeric value to each correctly scored item above the basal level until a ceiling is reached. The basal level is defined as the highest testing age equivalent at which the child scores all items correctly for two consecutive test ages. The ceiling is considered the highest test age at which the child scores any items correctly. An age equivalent is determined by adding the prescribed point value of each item scored correctly above the basal age to the basal age score. Therefore, if a child's basal score is 16 months, and he scores 1.5 points in the 18 month age set, 1 point in the 21 month age set and no points in the 24 month set, his age equivalent is 18.5 months.

THE DEVELOPMENTAL QUOTIENT

The developmental quotient is a concept of Gesell used to estimate a child's developmental level. Arithmetically, the DQ is calculated by dividing the child's age equivalent (AE) as determined by the means outlined above, by the child's chronological age (CA) and expressed as a percentage (see table III). A DQ is calculated for each of the language and visual motor scales separately and an average of these two DQs represents the overall level of function. The DQ, although not equivalent to an intelligence quotient, gives the clinician a reasonable estimate of a child's verbal and nonverbal cognitive abilities. The capacity to quantify the degree of delay by calculating the DQ provides the clinician with valuable information regarding the degree of delay, and pro-

Table III.   Developmental Quotient

DQ = Age Equivalent / Chronological Age X 100

A Neurodevelopmental Approach | 109

vides a useful tool in clarifying problems when counseling parents. It has already been mentioned that parents have a reasonably accurate estimation of their child's level of function by the time they present for evaluation. The Capute Scales provides the examiner and parents with objective information confirming the child's level of function in months, and the percentage of normal development present at the time of testing. To maximize confidence in the Capute Scale results, and to make sound inferences about future development, it is advisable to repeat the Capute Scales 6 to 12 months after the initial evaluation.

INTERPRETATION OF THE DEVELOPMENTAL QUOTIENTS

The interpretation of the developmental quotients employs the principals of delay, deviancy, and dissociation for formulating diagnoses. (See table IV.) Delay seen in cognitive, language, and visual motor scales, to a significant degree (DQ < 75), implies a diagnosis of mental retardation. Cognitive limitation must be accompanied by limited adaptive skills in order to make a formal diagnosis of mental retardation (AAMR). The child's family should be appropriately counseled about the suspicion of cognitive limitation, and when the timing seems prudent, referred for formal psychometric and adaptive testing.

Delay in the language domain of the Capute Scales that occurs in the presence of normal visual motor skills is indicative of a child with a communicative disorder or significant hearing loss, but normal cognition. In this case, the principles of delay and dissociation are used. The language stream is delayed and dissociates from a more normal developmental rate in the visual motor stream. Once language delay in the presence of normal cognition is established, hearing impairment must be ruled out, and further assessment of language ability is warranted. The language scale may be further scrutinized to look for a discrepancy (deviance or dissociation) between receptive and expressive abilities. Frequently it will be noted that a child understands language at an age appropriate level, commensurate with visual motor abilities, but expressive language is delayed. In mixed receptive and expressive language delay, both domains of language are less than expected for age or for visual motor abilities, but the two domains may not be equally depressed. It is not uncommon to see delayed receptive skills, with an even greater delay in expressive skills.

Table IV.   Capute Scales Interpretation

Language	Delayed	Delayed
Visual Motor	Delayed	Normal
Diagnosis	Mental Retardation	Developmental Language

Once a diagnosis of developmental language disorder is indicated by the Capute scale scoring, historical information and clinical observation of social skills and behavior are weighed to determine if the language delay is primary or a component of a broader developmental disorder such as autism or pervasive developmental disorder.

SUMMARY

Language delay in toddler and preschool age children is a common parental complaint. The first obligation of the clinician is to acknowledge the parent's concerns about delay and set out to assess the child thoroughly.

Assessment begins with a complete medical and developmental history to establish the nature and extent of delay, to assess historical risk for delay, which may indicate etiology, and to make assessment of progress in other streams of development. The physical examination that follows is concerned with identifying physical characteristics that may provide information regarding the etiology of the language delay. Neurological examination will rarely yield hard findings, but frequently will show softer neurological findings. The sum of the history and physical examinations direct the examiner to appropriate etiologic work-up considerations. In all cases of children with delayed language, a reliable hearing evaluation is essential.

Neurodevelopmental assessment to define the aspects of development that are abnormally affected entails the assessment of neuromotor findings, (primitive reflexes, postural reactions, and soft signs) as well as quantitative assessment of cognition and language and qualitative assessment of behavior, social, and adaptive skills, and pragmatics.

History, physical examination, medical work up, and hearing evaluations should rule out the majority of primary causes of language delay with the important exception of mental retardation. The quantitative measurement of abilities in the cognitive streams of language and visual motor skills is the key to differentiating mental retardation from a developmental language disorder in the child with language delay. There are numerous instruments available for the quantification of delay; therefore, the choice of instrument depends on the information required, the availability of time and appropriate evaluators, and the personal preference of the tester. In the primary care office, the Capute Scales are a reasonable choice for evaluation when information on both cognitive streams, and receptive and expressive skills are required. The benefits of the Capute Scales are four fold. The Capute scales quantify development in language and visual motor skills using the developmental quotient; require limited time, training, and instruments to administer; draw early expressive language information from parental history; and can provide information on language deviancy. Successful administration of the Capute Scales should distinguish the child with mental retardation from the child with isolated language delay. Qualitative observations during testing direct further evaluation after completion and interpretation of quantitative measures. A child with mental retardation will ultimately require referral for formal psychometric measures of intelligence and adaptive skills. A child with abnormal, stereotypic, or repetitive behaviors, and poor attempts at social interaction should have rating scales done for the autistic spectrum disorders. Finally children who, in the final analysis, are diagnosed with a primary developmental language disorder ought to be reviewed in the examiner's mind once more for problems frequently associated with language disorders, such as ADHD and behavioral problems.

Completion of the initial diagnostic evaluation of a language-delayed child is followed invariably with recommendations for appropriate management. The clinician must then think through intervention services that are warranted and make appropriate referrals. Some of the most frequently required services provided for language-delayed children are speech and language therapy and behavioral counseling. Developmental surveillance throughout the preschool years and into the early elementary school years is suggested to monitor progress and appropriateness of intervention as well as to monitor for associated learning difficulties.

REFERENCES

Accardo, P. J. 2002. Personal Communication.
American Association on Mental Retardation. 1992. *Mental Retardation: Definition, Classification, and Systems of Support, 9th ed.* Washington: American Association on Mental Retardation.
Bayley, N. 1969. *Bayley Scales of Infant Development.* New York: The Psychological Corporation.
Bayley, N. 1993. *Bayley Scales of Infant Development 2nd ed.* San Antonio: The Psychological Corporation.
Capute, A. J. 1996. *The Capute Scales: CAT/CLAMS Instruction Manual.* Baltimore.
Capute, A. J., Shapiro, B. K., Wachtel, R. C., Gunther, V. A., and Palmer, F. B. 1986. The Clinical Linguistic and Auditory Milestone Scale (CLAMS). *American Journal of Diseases of Childhood* 140:694–98.
Capute, A. J., Palmer, F., Shapiro, B. K., Wachtel, A., Schmidt, S., and Accardo, P. 1986. The Clinical Linguistic and Auditory Milestone Scale (CLAMS): Prediction of cognition in infancy. *Developmental Medicine and Child Neurology* 28:762–71.

Cattell, P. 1940. *The Measurement of Intelligence of Infants and Young Children.* New York: The Psychological Corporation.

Coplan, J. 1993. *Early Language Milestone Scale (2nd ed).* Austin, Texas: PRO-ED.

Dunn, L. M., and Dunn, L. M. 1997. *Peabody Picture Vocabulary Test, 3rd ed.* Circle Pines, MN: American Guidance Service.

Frankenburg, W. K., Dodds, J., Archer, P. et al. 1992. The Denver II: A major revision and restandardization of the Denver Developmental Screening Test. *Pediatrics* 89:91–97.

Gesell, A., and Amatruda, C. S. 1947. *Developmental Diagnosis Normal and Abnormal Child Development.* New York: Paul B. Hoeber.

Hoon, A. H., Pulsifer, M. G., Gopalan, R., Palmer, F. B., and Capute, A. J. 1993. The CAT/CLAMS in early cognitive assessment. *Journal of Pediatrics* 123: S1–S8.

Illingsworth, R. S. 1987. *The Development of the Infant and Young Child, Normal and Abnormal.* 9th ed. Edinburgh: Churchill Livingston.

Knobloch, H., and Pasamanick, B. (eds.) 1974. *Gesell and Amatruda's Developmental Diagnosis*, 3rd ed. Hagerstown: Harper & Row.

Kube, D. A., Wilson, W. M., Petersen, M. C., and Palmer, F. B. 2000. CAT/CLAMS: Its use in detecting early childhood cognitive impairments. *Pediatric Neurology* 23:208–15.

Leppert, M. L., Shank, T. P., Shapiro, B. K., and Capute, A. J. 1998. The Capute Scales: CAT/CLAMS—A pediatric assessment tool for the early detection of mental retardation and communicative disorders. *Mental Retardation and Developmental Disabilities Research Reviews* 4:14–19.

Lock, T. M., Shapiro, B. K., Ross, A., and Capute, A. J. 1986. Age of presentation in developmental disability. *Journal of Developmental and Behavioral Pediatrics* 7:340–45.

Pulsifer, M. B., Hoon, A. H., Palmer, F. B. et. al. 1994. Maternal estimates of developmental age in preschool children. *Journal of Pediatrics* 125:S18–S24.

Sheridan, M. 1964. Development of auditory attention and the use of language symbols. In *Clinics in Developmental Medicine No. 13: The Child Who Does Not Talk*, ed. C. Renfrew and K. Murphy. London, England. Spastics Society Medical Education and Information Unit with William Heinemann Medical Books Ltd.

Thorndike, R. K., Hagen, E. P., and Sattler, J. M. 1986. *The Stanford-Binet Intelligence Scale, 4th ed.* Chicago: Riverside Publishing Co.

Wachtel, R., Shapiro, B. K., Palmer, F. B., Allen, M. C., and Capute, A. J. 1994. CAT/CLAMS: A tool for the pediatric evaluation of infants and young children with developmental delay. *Clinical Pediatrics* 33:410–15.

Wachtel, R. C., Tepper, V. J., Houck, D., McGrath, C. J., and Thompson, C. 1994. Neurodevelopment in pediatrics HIV infection, the use of the CAT/CLAMS. *Clinical Pediatrics* 33:416–20.

Chapter 7

The Child Who Does Not Talk:
A Pediatric Overview

Pasquale J. Accardo

BACKGROUND

Parents tend to become concerned quickly at the slightest delay in ambulation as suggesting a significant motor delay. Thus the child who is not walking by 13 or 14 months is often brought to the pediatrician's attention and identified as a "late walker." In fact, the mean age for walking is closer to 13 months and not walking until 15 months represents only a minimal delay. Indeed, some otherwise perfectly normal children may not walk until much closer to their second birthday.

In contrast, it is not unusual to find children over two years of age who are not talking at all and whose parents view this situation as unremarkable. "He doesn't want to talk yet." "Einstein didn't talk until he was five years old." "The older children do all her talking for her." "He'll talk when he wants to." These and a variety of other pseudo-explanations are offered to rationalize a relative lack of concern for what are probably significant language delays. Such a laissez-faire attitude is reinforced by many physicians and non-medical professionals who share a voluntarist interpretation of the onset of speech and decline to view such a delay as needing attention.

Over the past two decades, professionals have emphasized the importance of early intervention, and the federal government and the states have funded programs to find and treat infants and young children with developmental delays. The successful identification of children with language delays in the first three years of life has required a major educational thrust aimed at both parents and professionals. The focus of this effort has been to emphasize the following:

- The development of communication skills in infants and young children proceeds in an orderly and sequential, and, therefore, predictable manner.
- Communication disorders are the most common developmental problem in early childhood (affecting an estimated 20% to 25% of all children) and so represent a significant portion of all developmental assessment and treatment services provided to children in this age group.
- Early diagnosis and early intervention for communication delays and disorders are accepted priorities in routine well child care provision.

The first two statements in combination seem to facilitate the early identification of such communication delays and disorders and so help to operationalize the third statement. Difficulties arise, however, from two major sources.

First, many professionals who deal with the routine developmental surveillance of infants and young children remain insufficiently familiar with the normal development of communication skills in such children. Indeed, there frequently persist misinterpretations of and myths about delays and disorders in this area that then act as barriers to appropriate service provision (table I).

Table I.   Myths About Language Delay

Communication is the same as spoken language.
Language cannot be assessed until the onset of spoken words.
Early diagnosis of communication delays and disorders cannot occur until after two years of age.
If communication delays and disorders could be diagnosed prior to age two, there are no effective interventions available.
The only markers for communication disorders in infancy and early childhood are specifically communication milestones.
Communication delays and disorders cannot be diagnosed under a year of age.

Second, despite the existing broad knowledge base on the development of communication skills in infancy and early childhood, the practical application of such information has serious limitations (table II).

Formal assessment of infant communication is thus fraught with pitfalls. None of the tests used approach the psychometric validity of similar tests used to assess communication in adults. The administration of infant tests often requires an experience of working with a wide range of children and of childhood disability patterns that belongs to few professionals. Despite these and similar limitations, assessment of infant language skills must be attempted if infants and

Table II.   Limitations in the Assessment of Communication Disorders in Infants and young Children

Many infant language tests are either poorly standardized or exhibit weak psychometric properties.

Many language instruments in use for infants and young children have an excessive reliance on parental report as opposed to direct observation.

Many assessments of communication skills in infants and young children take place outside the child's natural environment.

Many professionals have limited experience assessing communication skills in infants and very young children.

Many professionals involved in the assessment of communication disorders in infants and young children share in some or all of the myths described above.

young children with communication disorders are to be identified early and allowed to benefit from appropriate intervention. Formal screening needs to be routinely employed, and any observed delays should (almost) never be managed with a "wait and see" attitude.

CHILDREN AT RISK FOR COMMUNICATION DISORDERS

Even before a communication disorder is suspected, the presence of certain red flags, some directly reflecting communication skills and some indirectly associated with the presence of a communication disorder, should alert a child health professional to the possibility of a communication disorder (table III) and suggest a closer developmental surveillance.

Table III.   Red Flags for Communication Disorders in Children

Linguistic Red Flags for the Presence of a Communication Disorder

1. Quiet baby
2. Not talking
3. Poor speech intelligibility
4. Frustration with regard to communication
5. Echolalia
6. Limited vocabulary

Non-Linguistic Red Flags for the Presence of a Communication Disorder

7. Failure to thrive
8. Feeding disorders
9. Toe walking (persisting longer than three months)[1]
10. Severe temper tantrums
11. Attention deficit hyperactivity disorder
12. Abnormalities of tone in infancy including arching, non-cuddliness
13. Poor socialization skills

[1]Toe walking is one of those isolated autistic features that can also be used as a nonspecific marker for neurologically based communiation disorders (Accardo and Whitman 1989; Accardo et al. 1992)

Factors that place a child at risk for a hearing impairment (table IV) are a subset of medical factors that place a child at risk for a communication disorder (table V). It is interesting that recurrent otitis media does not appear to appreciably increase the risk for communication disorders in children (Lindsay et al. 1999).

Table IV.   Factors that Place a Child at Risk for Hearing Impairment

14.   Family history of hereditary childhood sensorineural hearing loss
15.   Congenital infections associated with hearing loss
16.   Craniofacial anomalies
17.   Birth weight under 1,500 gms.
18.   Hyperbilirubinemia requiring exchange transfusion
19.   Ototoxic medications
20.   Bacterial meningitis
21.   Apgar score of 0–4 at one minute or 0–6 at five minutes
22.   Mechanical ventilation support for 5 days or longer
23.   A syndrome known to include hearing loss.

(adapted from Joint Committee on Infant Hearing 1994)

Table V.   Medical Factors that Place a Child at risk for a Communication Disorder

24.   Prematurity[2]
25.   Recurrent/chronic otitis media
26.   Hearing impairment
27.   Microcephaly[3]
28.   Genetic disorders
29.   Feeding disorders, including failure to thrive
30.   Neurological/neurosurgical disorders affecting the brain
       a) cerebral palsy
       b) traumatic brain injury (TBI)
       c) microcephaly
       d) macrocephaly
       e) seizure disorder
       f) attention deficit hyperactivity disorder
31.   Lead poisoning
32.   Fetal alcohol syndrome
33.   Dysmorphic child
34.   Chronic illness/prolonged hospitalization, including tracheotomy
35.   Cleft lip/palate

[2]The more extreme the prematurity, the greater the risk for communication disorders and other developmental disabilities; the more complicated the perinatal course, the greater the risk for communication disorders and other developmental disabilities. Many genetic disorders that are associated with communication disorders are also associated with mental retardation or hearing impairment.

[3]Severe microcephaly tends to be associated with mental retardation. When, however, a child with microcephaly is not retarded, communication disorders represent a typical outcome. (Accardo and Whitman 1988).

There are a number of familial factors that may also heighten one's suspicion for the presence of a communication disorder (table VI). Signs and symptoms of feeding disorders (table VII) may be related to oral motor difficulties that will, in turn, affect articulation and language production later on. Isolated autistic features (table VIII) are also frequently associated with communication disorders: the more severe the language delay, the more a child without a diagnosis of autistic spectrum disorder will tend to exhibit some autistic features (Accardo 2000; for a more detailed description of screening, assessment, and diagnosis of autism, see Filipek et al. 1999, 2000).

Although it is useful to pay attention to these red flags for the presence of a communication disorder, many children with the above markers will not have communication disorders. Conversely, many children with communication disorders will not have any of the flagged conditions because most at risk children will not exhibit any

Table VI.   Familial Factors in Communication Disorders

36.	Family history of communication disorders, speech and language problems
37.	Parents with cognitive limitation
38.	Children in foster care
39.	Parents with hearing impairment
40.	Bilingual home environment
41.	Family history of child abuse, child neglect, child sexual abuse

Table VII.   Signs of Feeding Disorders Associated with Childhood Communication Disorders

42.	Poor weight gain
43.	Prolonged feeding time
44.	Poor suck
45.	Failure to thrive
46.	Craniofacial disorders/syndromes of the head and neck
47.	Gagging, choking
48.	Excessive drooling

Table VIII.   Isolated Autistic Features Associated with Childhood Communication Disorders

49.	Toe walking
50.	Poor eye contact
51.	Hand flapping
52.	Self stimulatory behavior (e.g., rocking, spinning)
53.	Acts as if deaf
54.	In own little world
55.	No peer interactions
56.	Arching
57.	Echoing

developmental disorders, and many children with developmental disorders will not have any risk factors.

Children with multiple red flags still seem to be at greater risk for the presence of a communication disorder. If an etiology has not been identified after a communication disorder is diagnosed, the same red flags become the primary list of considerations for differential diagnosis of an etiology.

ASSESSMENT OF THE CHILD WHO DOES NOT TALK

When a child presents with the suspicion of delayed communication skills, the evaluation must assess the severity of the delay to decide:

- whether the child meets criteria for the diagnosis of a communication disorder
- whether, even in the absence of the diagnosis of a disorder, the degree of delay indicates the appropriateness of some type of intervention
- the presence of a possible medical etiology for, or contribution to, the communication disorder
- the presence of some other risk factor or diagnosis that might qualify the child for some type of intervention.

The degree of delay may be described in terms of a language age, a language quotient, or a standard score. In infants and young children it is especially important to attempt to assess communication and language skills separately from non-verbal problem solving abilities. The Clinical Linguistic Auditory Milestones Scale (CLAMS, table IX) is an example of a brief screening instrument specifically developed for use in the pediatric office (Capute et al. 1981; Capute and Accardo 1996a, 1996b). It is important to note that the prospective assessment of infants and young children for the presence of a communication disorder involves no additional cost or significant investment of time. Simply asking several questions from a developmental checklist or using components of a standardized brief instrument at each well child visit will allow the professional to suspect a problem. Similarly the primary health care provider or early childhood professional should be accustomed to routinely observing important child/caregiver interactions.

A professional with the appropriate background, experience, and interest in the diagnosis of developmental disorders must then decide the extent of the biomedical evaluation appropriate to adequately pursue the identification of a specific etiology. On the one hand, the presence of certain genetic disorders can place an infant or young child at presumptive risk for the presence of a communication

Table IX.   Clinical Linguistic Auditory Milestones Scale (CLAMS)

6 wks	social smile	
3 mos	cooing	
4 mos	laughing	orient to mother's voice
5 mos	razzing/ah goo	orient to bell I
6 mos	babbling	
7 mos		orient to bell II
8 mos	dada/mama [non spec]	
9 mos	gesture	
10 mos	dada/mama [spec]	responds to "no"
12 mos	1 word	one step command with gesture
14 mos	3 words	
	immature jargoning	
16 mos	4 words	one step command without gesture
18 mos	6 words	points to one picture
		points to one body part
	vocabulary explosion	
22 mos	2 word phrases	
24 mos	50 words	points to a half dozen body parts
	2–3 word sentences	two step command
30 mos	pronouns	points to a half dozen pictures
3 years	3–4 word sentences	
4 years	4–5 word sentences	
5 years	5–6 word sentences	
6 years	6–7 word sentences	

(Modified from Capute and Accardo 1978).

disorder; on the other hand, the presence of a significant communication disorder should initiate the screening for genetic disorders associated with such communication patterns (table X). The possibility of a genetics consultation for a child with a communication disorder is increased in the presence of any of the following:

- Dysmorphic child
- Family history of developmental disabilities
- Severe communication disorder without other etiology
- Multiply handicapped child

Language is a complex phenomenon that does not readily lend itself to easy simplifications. However, instead of attempting to assess every possible influence on the development of language, the quality of infant communication, or the degree of normality, the physician should restrict himself or herself to distinguishing a significant degree of delay, and identifying the broad category of developmental disability.

The decision as to how far to pursue a specific etiology can be deferred to subspecialist consultants. To exemplify this process, the various patterns of language delay that can be seen in a two-year-old child will be reviewed. If a child presents at 24 months of age with no expressive

Table X.   Genetic Syndromes Associated with Communication Disorders

58. Angelman
59. Cornelia de Lange
60. Down
61. Duchenne muscular dystrophy
62. Fragile X
63. galactosemia
64. Rubinstein-Taybi
65. Klinefelter
66. sex chromosome aneuploidies
67. Smith-Magenis
68. tuberous sclerosis
69. Williams[4]

[4]Many of the conditions in this table (data from Udwin and Dennis 1995) are associated with significant cognitive impairment, but even in the presence of mental retardation, a child with one of these conditions often has a developmental profile with language skills noticeably worse than the level of general cognitive functioning. Children with Down syndrome have oral motor dysfunction contributing to articulation problems (a phonological disorder), recurrent otitis media contributing to hearing impairment, and also delayed expressive language skills on a neurogenetic basis. Non-verbal learning disabilities characterize many persons with fragile X syndrome and Turner syndrome. When isolated language skills are elevated (such as in Williams syndrome), they are often artificially inflated so that the child still has impaired language skills that would benefit from therapy. Such a child may score well on a specific test instrument, but the functional use of language remains below expectations.

language (no words), then the child's expressive language age is less than 12 months. This is automatically significant because the child's expressive language quotient is already below 50. One can try to close in further by assessing the presence of infant preverbal vocalizations and gesture usage. A child with a severe expressive language delay may have:

- An isolated expressive language delay/disorder
- A communication disorder with both expressive and receptive language delays
- Mental retardation (global developmental delay)
- An autistic spectrum disorder
- Hearing impairment

If the two-year-old child with expressive language delay has intact receptive language for age, then mental retardation is ruled out. There are several excellent receptive milestones that come in between 18 and 24 months of age to help quantify the child's receptive abilities: starting at about 18 months of age, children will begin to point to one body part and one picture in a book; by 24 months they will be able to point to many body parts and many pictures. An alternative milestone that is not typically very useful is the ability to follow one and two step commands. The difficulty with this milestone is that one step commands come in at about one year of age while two step commands come in nearer to two years of age. If the child follows one step commands but not two step commands, the examiner does not know just where between one and two years of age the child's receptive abilities lie. Perhaps this child will begin to follow two step commands at 25 months. Indeed, many children in the negativistic "terrible two's" are not receptive to any commands on a developmental-behavioral basis. When receptive language is intact, it is unlikely that hearing represents a significant contributing factor. However, it is standard practice to obtain formal audiological assessment on any child who exhibits language delay with any pattern.

An isolated expressive language delay is the single most common developmental problem in children. It can be divided into two major categories: (1) slow talkers, and (2) neurologically based developmental disorders of expressive language. Because the first group will exhibit a delay that typically corrects itself within less than a year (Paul 1991), it is debatable whether they really need any therapy. The problem is that there are no clear criteria to distinguish to which of these two groups a child with an expressive language delay belongs. Two possible approaches to discriminate the subgroup of isolated expressive language disorders can be suggested:

First, the child with expressive language delay who has one or more of the following probably has a neurologically based disorder of expressive language that would benefit from intervention:

- Prematurity
- Toe walking
- A family history of language disorders
- Oral motor difficulties
- Failure to thrive
- Microcephaly
- Echolalia
- A genetic syndrome

The child with none of these findings is more likely a slow talker.

Alternately, a second approach to the two-year-old child with delayed expressive language involves encouraging language stimulating experiences (such as a play group with other toddlers who are already talking) and then reevaluating after three months. If expressive language demonstrates a significant spurt forward, the child is probably a slow talker; if minimal progress occurs, then a neurologically based language disorder can be suspected.

If the child is shown to have receptive abilities as delayed as expressive abilities, then the developmental differential diagnosis becomes one between communication disorder and mental retardation. In order to make this discrimination an infant psychological test to tap non-verbal abilities is required. If non-verbal intelligence is intact, then the child has a communication disorder; if non-verbal intelligence is delayed, then the child may be mentally retarded or globally delayed. In the absence of such formal psychometrics, the child's non-verbal cognition can be estimated by asking the parent about the child's preferred form of interaction with toys. The levels of interaction can be briefly described as follows:

- Visual tracking   0–3 months
- Grasping   3–6 months
- Mouthing   6–9 months
- Banging/noisemaking   9–12 months
- Casting release [includes
  receptacle play]   12–15 months
- Stacking blocks   15–18 months
- Pieces in puzzle board   18–21 months
- Scribbling with crayon   21–24 months

Although these developmental levels are very approximate, the two-year-old child who still predominantly mouths toys can be considered significantly delayed, while the two-year-old child who is solving several-piece inset puzzles probably has intact non-verbal intelligence.

That leaves autism to be considered in the differential diagnosis. Confusing the picture is the fact that more than half of children with autism are also mentally retarded. Nevertheless, a child with an autistic spectrum disorder will present with one of three expressive language patterns: no expressive language, delayed expressive language, or apparently normal expressive language milestones.

The expressive language milestones expected for the typical two-year-old child include a vocabulary of at least 50 words, and the use of 2- or 3-word spontaneous phrases/beginning sentences. Some children with autistic spectrum disorder will appear to achieve both these milestones. It is, however, important to distinguish between the spontaneous use of words and phrases and the echoing (repeating in a robotic or non-communicative fashion) of such words and phrases. Children with autism sometimes exhibit the paradoxical language profile of expressive language skills being in advance of receptive language skills. This can only occur when the advanced expressive "language" is actually non-communicative in intent.

Autistic spectrum disorders involve both disordered communication and problems with socialization. Two excellent markers for autism in a two year child are (1) the absence of pretend play, and (2) the absence of joint attention. Pretend play involves the use of objects for make-believe such as pouring imaginary tea from a toy teapot and then drinking from the empty cup. One example of joint attention involves a third use of pointing:

- Children point to something they want (demand pointing)
- Children point to identify something (naming pointing)
- Children point to something that they want to share their interest in with another (protodeclarative pointing)

CONCLUSION

A comprehensive developmental language screening in young children can be accomplished by obtaining expressive and receptive language ages from an instrument such as the CLAMS, a parental description of the child's preferred interaction with toys, and ascertaining the presence of echoing, pretend play and joint attention.

The whole differential screening process can be accomplished in less than ten minutes and is thus within the reach of every primary care child health professional.

REFERENCES

Accardo, P. J. (Panel Chairman) et al. 1999a. *Clinical Practice Guideline: Report of the Recommendations: Communication Disorders, Assessment and Intervention for Young Children (Age 0–3 Years).* Albany, New York: New York State Department of Health. [Publication No. 4218]

Accardo, P. J. (Panel Chairman) et al. 1999b. *Clinical Practice Guideline: Quick Reference Guide: Communication Disorders, Assessment and Intervention for Young Children (Age 0–3 Years).* Albany, New York: New York State Department of Health. [Publication No. 4219]

Accardo, P. J. (Panel Chairman) et al.1999c. *Clinical Practice Guideline: The Guideline Technical Report: Communication Disorders, Assessment and Intervention for Young Children (Age 0–3 Years).* Albany, New York: New York State Department of Health. [Publication No. 4220]

Accardo, P. J. 2000. Diagnostic issues in autism. In *Autism: Clinical and Research Issues,* eds. P. J. Accardo, C. Magnusen, and A. J. Capute. Baltimore: York Press.

Accardo, P. J., and Whitman, B. Y. 1988. Severe microcephaly with normal non-verbal intelligence. *Pediatric Reviews and Communications* 3:61–65.

Accardo, P. J., and Whitman, B. Y. 1989. Toe walking: A marker for language disorders in the developmentally disabled. *Clinical Pediatrics* 28:347–50.

Accardo, P. J., Morrow, J., Heaney, M. S., Whitman, B. Y., and Tomazic, T. 1992. Toe walking and language development. *Clinical Pediatrics* 1:158–60.

Capute, A. J., and Accardo, P. J. 1978. Linguistic and auditory milestones in the first two years of life: A language inventory for the practicing pediatrician. *Clinical Pediatrics* 17:847–53.

Capute, A. J., and Accardo, P. J. 1996a. The infant neurodevelopmental assessment: A clinical interpretive manual for CAT-CLAMS in the first two years of life. Part 1. *Current Problems in Pediatrics* 26:238–57.

Capute, A. J., and Accardo, P. J. 1996b. The infant neurodevelopmental assessment: A clinical interpretive manual for CAT-CLAMS in the first two years of life. Part 2. *Current Problems in Pediatrics* 26:279–306.

Capute, A. J., Palmer, F. B., Shapiro, B. K., Wachtel, R. C., and Accardo, P. J. 1981. Early language development: clinical application of the Language and Auditory Milestones Scale. In *Language Behavior in Infancy and Early Childhood*, ed. R.E. Stark. New York: Elsevier-North Holland.

Filipek, P. A., Accardo, P. J., Baranek, G. T., Cook, E. H., Jr., Dawson, G., Gordon, B., Gravel, J. S., Johnson, C. P., Kallen, R. J., Levy, S. E., Minshew, N. J., Prizant, B. M., Rapin, I., Rogers, S. J., Stone, W. L., Teplin, S., Tuchman, R. F., and Volkmar, F. R. 1999. The screening and diagnosis of autistic spectrum disorders. *Journal of Autism and Developmental Disorders* 29:437–82.

Filipek, P. A., Accardo, P. J., Ashwal, S., Baranek, G. T., Cook, E. H., Jr., Dawson, G., Gordon, B., Gravel, J. S., Johnson, C. P., Kallen, R. J., Levy, S. E., Minshew, N. J., Ozonoff, S., Johnson, C. P., Prizant, B. M., Rapin, I., Teplin, S., Rogers, S. J., Stone, W. L., Tuchman, R. F., and Volkmar, F. R. 2000. Practice parameter: Screening and diagnosis of autism: Report of the Quality Standards Subcommittee of the American Academy of Neurology and the Child Neurology Society. *Neurology* 55:468–79.

Joint Committee on Infant Hearing. 1994. Position statement. *Pediatrics* 95:152–56.

Lindsay, R. L., Tomazic, T., Whitman, B. Y., and Accardo, P. J. 1999. Early ear problems and developmental problems at school age. *Clinical Pediatrics* 38:123–32.

Paul, R. 1991. Profiles of toddlers with slow expressive language development. *Topics in Language Disorders* 11:1–13.

Udwin, O., and Dennis, J. 1995. Psychological and behavioural phenotypes in genetically determined syndromes: A review of research findings. In *Behavioural Phenotypes*, eds. G. O'Brien and W. Yule. London: Mac Keith Press.

Chapter • 8

Neuroimaging and Disorders of Communication

*William Davis Gaillard, Ben Xu, and
Lyn Balsamo*

This chapter reviews the use of functional imaging to elucidate the organization of language processing networks in children during development and in disease states. To appreciate the capacities and limitations of functional imaging, the chapter begins with a brief review of functional imaging principles. This is followed by a consideration of imaging language in normal children and then in children with neurological conditions, principally epilepsy, but also stroke, and will only briefly touch upon the rapidly expanding imaging experience in learning and reading disabilities. Children have a tremendous capacity for recovery for language functions following acute and focal brain insult. This chapter will provide the imaging evidence for where that recovery occurs and presents the view that language capacity is restricted to certain brain regions, though plasticity of language functions within these areas persists, with diminishing degrees, into adolescence.

FUNCTIONAL NEUROIMAGING PRINCIPLES

Functional neuroimaging with radioactive tracers, as used in 15O water PET, or with functional MRI (fMRI), relies on the observation that local increases in neuronal activity are associated with regionally specific and tightly regulated increases in blood flow. Most fMRI investigations use a blood oxygen level dependent (BOLD) imaging technique. Functional MRI detects the changes in MRI signal that are

associated with increased blood flow that principally result from increase in the oxyhemoglobin /deoxyhemoglobin ratio seen with the
luxury hyperperfusion beyond immediate physiologic need (see
Cohen et al. 1994; Moonen and Bandettini 2000). The spatial resolution
for most fMRI is 3 to 4 mm, for whole brain acquisition, but to enhance signal to noise with smoothing techniques resolution is often reduced to 8 to 9 mm. Resolution of 1 to 2 mm is possible when imaging
restricted brain regions. The temporal resolution is linked to the timing of the hemodynamic response that occurs 2 to 4 seconds after
stimulus and reaches a peak at 4 to 8 seconds (Malonek et al. 1997).
The bulk of the hemodynamic response is derived from synaptic activity (Logothetis et al. 2001).

Functional MRI studies are conducted by serially imaging the
brain while a task is performed. Experimental paradigms compare signals in brain regions between two or more conditions. Most paradigms employ a boxcar design using a control and experimental
condition. Semi automated programs are employed to screen the data
set for differences in signal between conditions. Areas that exceed the
statistical threshold are then flagged as a red or yellow pixel and
deemed "activated." Activated areas may be identified on the raw
functional images, or overlaid on a higher resolution image. Although
it is more pleasing to view maps on the higher resolution anatomical
studies, the resolution is less than when viewing the raw images.

As a consequence, fMRI methods are indirect measures of brain
activity. They measure relative changes in neuronal activity; they rely
heavily on choice of paradigm that results in both initiating the hemodynamic response and assuring that there is significant change in
blood flow between experimental and control conditions. Such methods can only identify areas involved in a given task; they cannot
determine whether they are critical to it—for instance, circuits implicated in attention are seen during many language tasks. Some critical
areas may not be identified because a sufficient hemodynamic response was not initiated—as may be seen if the task is too simple—or
because control and task conditions are indistinct. Temporal resolution is well beyond the firing and conduction rates of neurons (msec).
Thus the networks involved in the task may be identified, but the timing and interplay between regions may not be elucidated—such methods are only possible with real time measures of neuronal activity
such as magneto-electroencephalography, but they are limited in the
sophistication of the paradigms possible (Breier et al. 2001). Recent advances in MR technology allow quantitative blood flow measures (Ye
et al. 1998; Lia et al. 2000) with arterial spin tagging techniques.

Tasks must be adapted for cognitive ability in pediatric or patient populations. Choice of experimental conditions is particularly

important as control conditions commonly used for adults may be interpreted as language in younger children thus obscuring activation signal. For example, language areas involved in reading processing may be used to determine whether pseudowords, letter strings, or false fonts—all commonly used as control conditions in adult reading studies—are real words. Unmonitored covert studies are often performed because they minimize motion. Covert responses and push button responses provide task performance monitoring, but may increase motion artifact and add an additional layer of cognitive processing that complicates data interpretation.

Most investigators report results as a group analysis in a standard (adult) anatomic atlas. Commonly employed analysis programs interrogate data sets in a standard brain atlas (spatial normalization) in order to enhance signal to noise, and to employ probability methods to test applicability to wider populations. As a consequence individual variability is lost. This is an important limitation for investigation of disease states, such as epilepsy, or learning disorders, such as dyslexia, where heterogeneity is the rule. An advantage of fMRI is the ability to obtain individual maps that can be used to establish variability or be compared to group "normal" maps. Such methods have proved useful in identifying language networks in children and adults with chronic epilepsy to plan surgical resection.

Functional MRI relies on the ability of children to remain still and cooperate with the task. Most pediatric studies report on children eight and older. The youngest age of reported activation maps for cognitive tasks is five years, though some children as young as four may be studied, but these are unusual and may introduce a greater subject selection bias. There are also particular challenges to imaging children both from the technical aspects of image acquisition and paradigm design. These issues have recently been reviewed (Bookheimer et al. 2000; Gaillard, Grandin, and Xu 2001). The BOLD response appears to be similar in adults and children (Gaillard, Grandin, and Xu 2001). Investigators, however, often find a need to use varying thresholds in children and in pediatric patients.

FUNCTIONAL MRI STUDIES OF LANGUAGE ORGANIZATION IN NORMAL CHILD POPULATIONS

There are an increasing number of studies conducted in children using fMRI. They include language studies (described below), visual spatial processing (Pugliese 1999), face recognition (Nelson et al. 2000; Thomas et al. 2001), attention (Vaidya et al. 1998), and working memory (Casey et al. 1995, Casey et al. 1997; Thomas et al. 1999). These studies show that activation patterns are fundamentally the same in children as in adults for the ages studied, mostly seven and above. This section will concentrate on language studies that include verbal fluency, semantic decision, auditory comprehension, and reading processing (see figure 1).

The most widely studied tasks are those of verbal fluency—such as generating a verb from either a noun (Schlagger 2001) or from categories (both semantic tasks) (Gaillard, Grandin, and Xu 2001), or generating words that begin with a letter (a phonemic task) (Gaillard, Hertz-Pannier, Mott et al. 2000; Gaillard, Grandin, and Xu 2001). Other tasks require semantic decisions, such as determining whether two words are in the same category (Serafani et al. 2001). The clues may be auditory or visual. As a rule, the above mentioned tasks are strong activators of the frontal lobe language processing areas that lie in inferior and mid frontal cortex (dorsolateral prefrontal cortex, Brodmann Areas (BA) 44, 45, 46, 47, 9) (For adult review see Thompson-Schill et al. 1997; Poldrack et al. 1999). The activation is strongly, but not completely, lateralized to the left language dominant hemisphere. Activation patterns for all these fluency and decision tasks are similar. Studies in normal children show fundamentally similar activation to adults, principally in left inferior frontal gyrus (IFG) but also in mid frontal gyrus (MFG) (figures 2 and 3). There is variable activation in temporal lobe on an individual basis because of the low cognitive burden of the receptive aspects of the tasks. Some studies suggest that activation in younger children is more extensive or more bilateral than adults in IFG (Gaillard, Hertz-Pannier, Mott et al. 2000; Holland et al. 2001), but other studies find less extensive activation, but similar laterality than adults (Gaillard, Grandin, and Xu 2001). It is likely that some of these discrepancies may be explained by technical issues pertaining to pediatric imaging, and the small number of younger children studied (Gaillard, Grandin, and Xu 2001). Additional activation is typically seen in anterior cingulate gyrus and supplementary motor area. These regions are implicated in attention and motor planning of the response, but are not critical to language processing itself.

Paradigms that place a demand on receptive processing identify the dominant temporal area, Wernicke's area, involved in language processing. Reading tasks that involve a written text, in contrast to single words, show consistent and strong activation in left middle and superior temporal gyrus (BA 21, 22) (figures 2 and 3) (adult studies: Just et al. 1996; Bevalier et al. 1997; children: Gaillard, Pugliese, Grandin et al. 2001). There is additional activation in left fusiform gyrus, likely from word form identification (Gaillard, Pugliese, Grandin et al. 2001; see Pugh et al. 1996). Frontal activation is seen in BA 44, 45, and 9, and again likely have to do with working memory

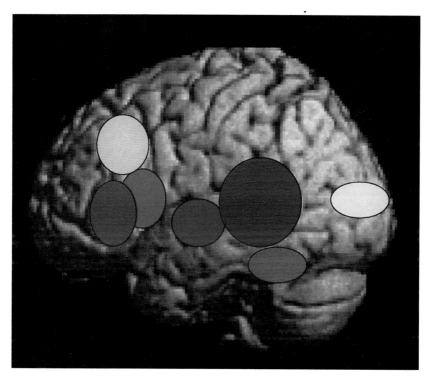

Figure 1. Schematic for language processing areas in left, dominant hemi-sphere showing primary and auditory cortex (blue) (bilateral); primary and second order visual cortex (white) bilateral; inferior temporal cortex (fusiform and lingual gyrus) for letter feature identification (orange); "Wernicke's Area": semantic processing areas that derive meaning from written and spo-ken word (red). Broca's Area: planning speech (green), involved in all fluency and recall studies; areas involved in semantic decision (pink); areas involved in verbal working memory (yellow).

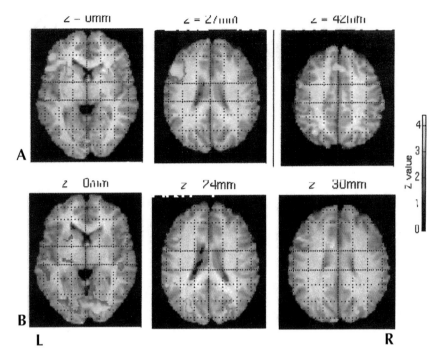

Figure 2.   SPM group activation maps in adults for: A: covert verbal fluency to categories compared to rest (29, mean age 28 years) and B: reading fables compared to a visual dot control (21, mean age 27 years).
"Activated" areas (random effect, $p < 0.05$). Shown in yellow, orange, and red (z score). Left image is left brain.

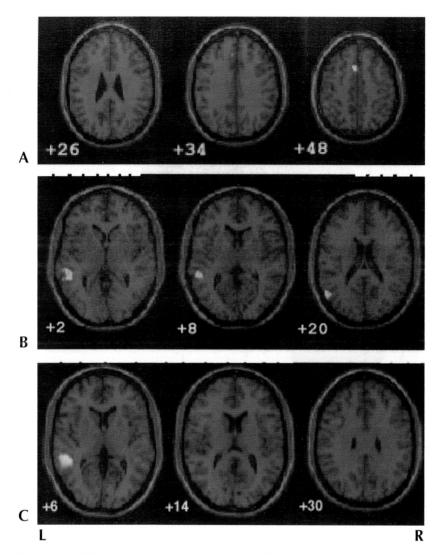

Figure 3.   SPM group activation maps for children: A: covert verbal fluency to categories compared to rest (14 children, 8–12 years, mean age 10.2 years); B: Listening to stories compared to reverse speech control (16 children, 5–7.9 years, mean age 7.1 years); and C: reading fables compared to a visual dot control (12 children, 5–7.9 years, mean age 72. years). Left image is left brain.

Reading Three-Letter Words

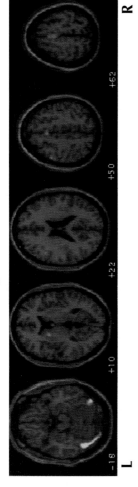

Figure 4. SPM group maps for young children reading 3 letter single words; 6 children range 6.5–7.0 years old (mean 6.6). Left image is left brain.

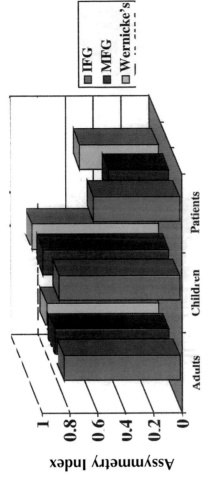

Figure 5. 3D graph showing AI for a read response naming task (reading a 5–6 word sentence that describes an object, e.g., "what is a long yellow fruit?") in normal children (mean age 10 yr), normal adults (mean 28 yr), and patients (pediatric and adult) demonstrating the decreased AI in patients which results from increased right hemispheric activation.

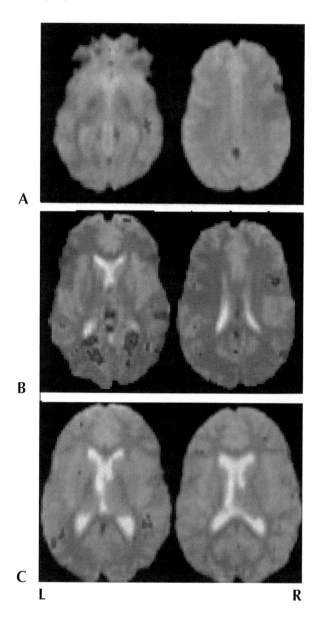

A

B

C

L   R

Figure 6.   Reading a fable in a 7 year old; activation maps at varying thresholds showing activation in homologous regions in right, non-dominant hemisphere. This finding is common in adults and children. A, $t = 5$; B, $t = 4$; c, $t = 3$. Left image is left brain.

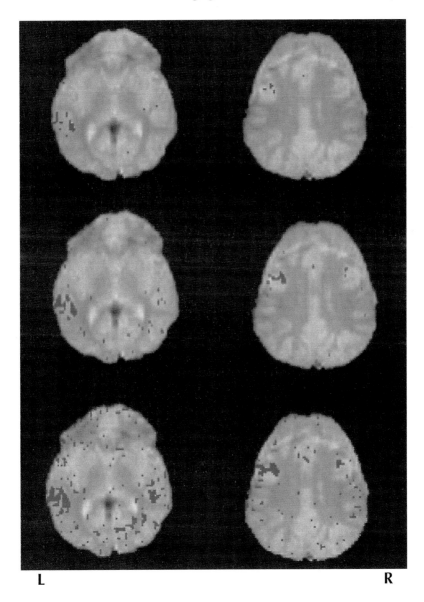

L **R**

Figure 7. Patients with left temporal lobe epilepsy showing atypical activation, all in right hemisphere in homologous regions. Tasks include A: verbal fluency; B: auditory response naming (naming to a 5 word description of an object, control rest); C: read response naming. All patients were right hemisphere dominant for language confirmed by IAT and surgery (t maps, $t = 4.0$). Left image is left brain.

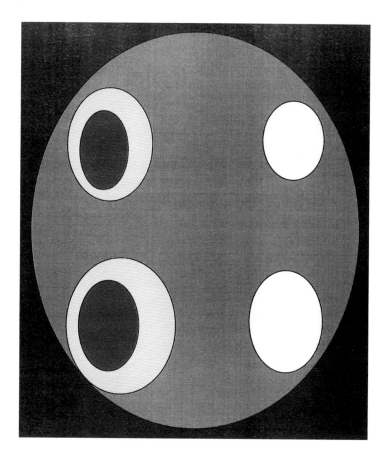

Figure 8. Proposed model for location of language processing. Red, normal left dominant activation. Light yellow, activation in children with early onset brain injury, shifted to homologous regions in right hemisphere. Dark yellow, reorganization of language function to margins of typical language areas, in children with later (or less severe) insult.

and grammatical decision (Gaillard, Pugliese, Grandin et al. 2001; Dapretto and Bookheimer 1999). As with adults, more grammatically complex text also elicits some right homologous temporal activation (Gaillard, Pugliese, Grandin et al. 2001; Just et al. 1996). The activation patterns for reading sentences and stories is the same for literate children as young as five and adults where activation is highly lateralized and regionally specific. Activation patterns for reading in early literate children, compared to more skilled readers, shows greater activation in fusiform, IFG (BA 44), premotor/motor and supplementary motor areas. Activation in these children is neither diffuse nor widespread, rather it is focal and regionally specific, which suggests a phonological strategy for early readers (age 6, personal observations, figure 4).

A limitation of reading studies is their applicability to pre- or non-literate populations. Furthermore, language is primarily an auditory phenomenon. Tasks that require auditory comprehension, such as listening to stories (adults: Mazoyer et al. 1993; Schlosser et al. 1998; children: Ulualp et al. 1998; Ahmad et al. 2001), naming based on a description of an object (adults: Bookheimer et al. 1997, 1998; children: Balsamo et al. 2002), or deciding whether a sentence makes syntactic sense (Booth et al. 1999, 2000) engage cortex along the middle and posterior aspect of the superior temporal sulcus. Patterns in children are again strongly regionally specific and, with the proper control, highly lateralized. An auditory naming task, without an auditory control, shows activation in left and right superior temporal gyrus with greater activation seen on the left (by about 50%, but less marked than fluency or reading paradigms) that extend to posterior superior temporal gyrus (STG) and inferior parietal gyrus (BA 21, 22, 39). The naming aspect of the task elicits activation in superior left IFG and MFG. These naming tasks are reliable in children to age seven (Balsamo et al. in press). Listening to stories, without an auditory control condition, yields similar findings in temporal cortex but weak lateralization (Ulualp et al. 1998). These two auditory based naming and listening tasks did not account for primary auditory, and some second order auditory processing that is bilateral. When a reverse speech foil is used, which "controls" for early auditory processing, the regions for language processing are clearly seen to be regionally specific in the left superior sulcus extending to supramarginal gyrus on the left, as has been shown in adults (Schlosser et al. 1998; Mazoyer et al. 1993; Lehericy et al. 2000) and in children as young as 5 to 7 years old (Ahmad et al. 2001) (figure 3).

Minor differences in activation maps between adults and children most likely reflect skill and strategy employed for the task, rather than differences or diffuseness in neural networks themselves. All adults and children exhibit some degree of activation in homologous areas of non-dominant hemisphere, that is also more pronounced with increased task difficulty. It is unclear what non-dominant activation contributes to language processing. These areas may play an important role in supporting plasticity of language organization in the setting of brain injury, discussed below (figure 7).

PATIENT POPULATIONS AND LANGUAGE REORGANIZATION

The premise of fMRI as a tool that can successfully identify brain regions involved in neural processing has been confirmed in epilepsy and tumor populations. These patients commonly undergo surgical resection of their seizure focus or their tumor. Intra-carotid amytal tests (IAT) are performed to determine the hemisphere dominant for language before surgery, and many patients undergo electrical cortical stimulation (ECS) to delineate language areas in relation to the seizure focus or tumor in an effort to spare essential functions. This population provides a means to compare fMRI methods with IAT and ECS. Comparisons with verbal fluency and semantic decision tasks are excellent in adults, and children (adults: Demb et al. 1995; Binder et al. 1996; Yetkin et al. 1998; Benson et al. 1999; Lehericy et al. 2000; Fernandez et al. 2001; Billingsley et al. 2001; Binder et al. 2002; children: Hertz-Pannier et al. 1997; Stapleton et al. 1997; Harvey et al. 1999; Logan et al. 1999; Keene et al. 2000). Auditory naming tasks and reading tasks also show excellent agreement (Hunter et al. 1999; Gaillard, Bookheimer, and Cohen 2000, Gaillard, Balsamo, Grandin et al. 2000, Graillard, Balsamo, Xu et al. 2001).

However, approximately 5% of patient studies show some form of incomplete disagreement: one method is lateralized while the other indicates bilateral dominance. Rare cases of complete disagreement can be found where functional imaging methods were correct (Pardo and Fox 1993; Hunter et al. 1999) or where IAT was correct (Gaillard, Bookheimer, and Cohen 2000). In the latter circumstances large tumors or vascular malformations may alter the BOLD response (Gaillard, Bookheimer, and Cohen 2000). Electrical cortical stimulation shows very good but not complete agreement with localization, as most occur within one cm of each other (Bookheimer et al. 1997; Fitzgerald et al. 1997). For both ECS and IAT some discrepancies may reflect differences in test paradigms utilized that make direct comparison problematic. For instance most IAT and ECS rely heavily on object naming, a task that has been unreliable in individual fMRI patient application (Benson et al. 1999). For ECS and IAT, technical factors may also account for some differences: the bulk of BOLD signal occurs in draining veins millimeters remote from primary involved regions, and image distortion inherent in fast imaging techniques and from co-registration. Finally, it should also be recalled that not all areas identified by fMRI are critical to task performance, and not all critical areas may be identified. For these reasons a panel of tasks is employed to identify various networks involved in language processing.

A previous chapter has shown that children retain a remarkable capacity to recover language functions in the setting of brain injury, mostly stroke, tumor, and traumatic brain injury. When injury is acute and focal, in contrast to prolonged global ischemic injury, recovery is possible. Children affected at earlier ages may experience a complete recovery. Recent work has shown that the capacity for meaningful recovery extends into early adolescence, suggesting plasticity for language function is great. Functional MRI provides a means to discern where that recovery occurs, and has been performed with this view in pediatric epilepsy and stroke populations.

Adults with epilepsy of childhood onset have a higher likelihood of atypical language that cannot be predicted on the basis of anatomy alone. IAT, and recently fMRI, has shown that patients with early onset of epilepsy or brain injury are more likely to have altered language representation. Children with left hemispheric injury before age two who are left handed have an 80% chance of bilateral or right hemispheric dominance for speech. These studies do not discern whether epilepsy or an antecedent remote cause is the driving force.

Intra-carotid amytal test in epilepsy patients has shown that 4% of right handed individual are right hemisphere dominant; in contrast, 30% of left handers have left or bilateral language. If there is a history of early left hemisphere insult, then 20% of right handers and 80% of left handers show bilateral or right hemisphere dominance (Rasmussen and Milner 1977; Woods, Eodrill, and Ojemann 1988). Intra-carotid amytal test provides laterality, but not localization, of speech functions. Electrical cortical stimulation studies show atypical location of language disruption in left hemisphere (Ojemann et al. 1989; Devinsky et al. 1993). Although intra-hemispheric variability is found, normal variability for these functions is not known for comparison. Functional imaging in adults recapitulates IAT and ECS findings. Pujol et al. (1999) compared MFG activation during word fluency and measures of left handedness. They found 4% of right handed individuals had right dominance, and 20% of left handers had right or bilateral speech. Atypical language activation occurred in homologous areas in the right hemisphere. Springer et al. (1999) compared 50 adult patients with epilepsy to 100 normal adult controls using an auditory based semantic decision task (whether the task item was found in North America and useful to humans). They used hemispheric laterality indices, and found 4% right handers were right or bilateral language dominant. They did not look at regional activation. They found that 22% of their patients had bilateral or right language dominance, nearly all of whom had epilepsy onset before age six years. They did not comment on structural abnormalities nor did they distinguish between epilepsy or remote injury as the cause for reorganized language networks.

Müller et al. (1999) studied eleven individuals (including two 8-year-olds and five teenagers) with left-hemisphere lesions and nine normal adults. Using ^{15}O-water-PET they found evidence for a shift to right hemisphere lateralization for some language functions in those with early onset epilepsy. Leftward asymmetry of activation was strongly reduced in an early onset group ($\leq$ 6 years, n = 6) as compared to a late onset group (n = 5) and normal controls. These differences approached significance in the inferior frontal and superior temporal regions for receptive language tasks; however, they met significant levels in the prefrontal, inferior frontal, and inferior parietal regions for the expressive task (sentence repetition). Rightward shifts among the early onset group were a result of enhanced activation in the right hemisphere, in addition to reduced activation in the lesional left hemisphere. In contrast, Loring et al. (1999), in reviewing IAT in 561 patients with left temporal lobe epilepsy and did not find a difference in age of epilepsy onset (age 9) between left and anomalous dominant patients.

We have performed fMRI language paradigms on 51 adult and pediatric patients with refractory partial epilepsy (24 children aged 7–16 years and 27 adults aged 17 to 55) and compared results to IAT and ECS in 36 patients (Hertz-Pannier et al. 1997; Gaillard et al. 2002; Gaillard, Bookheimer, and Cohen 2000; Gaillard, Xu, Balsamo et al. 2000; Gaillard and Theodore 2000; Gaillard, Balsamo, Xu et al. 2001). We employed a panel of tasks to assess verbal fluency, reading comprehension, auditory comprehension, and semantic recall. All individual data sets were analyzed using a region of interest analysis on individual t maps to identify frontal and temporal regional activation. In our fMRI studies, ten of the 51 (aged 7 to 55 years) patients were left handed or ambidextrous, and four of those ten had atypical language representation. Of the 41 right-handers, 7 (17%) have right or bilateral language representation. In contrast 3% to 4% of our normal volunteer studies have atypical language (χ^2 < 0.001). The children with atypical language representation ranged in age of seizure onset from 0.5 to 12 years; six were younger than seven, two of whom had early (< 2 years) focal left hemispheric insult. Furthermore, the degree of asymmetry for IFG, MFG, and Wernicke's regions were significantly lower among patients mostly due to increased right hemisphere activation (figure 5) (Gaillard, Balsamo, Xu et al. 2001). All bilateral or right activation occurred in homologous brain areas in the right hemisphere (figure 6).

There is some evidence from IAT that some patients have mixed rather than bilateral dominance (Kurthen 1992). The latter phenomenon was also observed in a group of patients with congenital right hemiparesis caused by unilateral lesions in the left anterior periventricular white matter (Staudt et al. 2001). Staudt and his colleagues used fMRI and expressive (word generation) and receptive (listening to story) tasks to identify language processing cortex. They found that during language production, patients showed a shift in activation to the frontal lobe of the undamaged right hemisphere proportional to the degree of frontal periventricular white matter injury. In contrast, activation corresponding to language reception remained in the left temporal lobe. Right frontal activation was in homologous regions. The authors hypothesized that damage to the motor tracts controlling speech output prompted a shift in dominance. These findings may help explain shifts in language and hand dominance among those with an epileptic focus in the frontal lobe (Rasmussen and Milner 1977; Woods, Dodrill, and Ojemann 1988), and highlight the importance of paradigm selection and regional analysis. Another study examining premature children found that those who were extremely premature had imaging evidence for more extensive ischemic injury, and those who were cognitively impaired showed activation patterns that implicate a phonemic strategy for a task designed to identify semantic processing networks (Peterson personal communication). In light of our experience with reading in younger children, these findings suggest reliance on developmentally less mature but capable networks.

Booth et al. (1999, 2000) studied six pediatric patients with perinatal strokes or periventricular hemorrhages (five in left hemisphere, one in right) in comparison to seven typical children and five adults. They utilized a paradigm in which children were required to listen to sentences that varied in syntactic complexity (children responded to a true/false question identifying the subject of the sentence). Asymmetry indices were calculated by hemisphere and by regions of interest. Healthy children and adults activated a left hemisphere pattern including superior temporal, middle temporal, inferior frontal, prefrontal, and anterior central sulcus regions. They found that the patient group activated a similar pattern in the right hemisphere.

There are competing views on the brain's ability to compensate for language representation in the face of injury. One view maintains the early childhood brain is pluripotent and that extensive brain areas can sustain language function in response to injury. The alternative view maintains that language function is programmed to be sustained by discretely defined and specific brain regions, with restricted capacity for reorganization constrained by a critical period that may extend into late childhood and early adolescence (Lennenberg 1967; Bates et al. 1997; Bates 1999). A clue to our understanding of brain plasticity comes from imaging data. Functional MRI data from patients with epilepsy and in patients with perinatal or neonatal ischemia and stroke shows variability in language organization, but always confined to homologous areas in right hemisphere. Activation patterns in the above studies appear confined to classical language areas and are restricted in location.

Another clue to the phenomena of language network plasticity can be found in adult and child normal volunteer studies. Some degree of right activation is seen for all tasks—ranging from 10% to 35%—and becomes more apparent at "less rigorous" t thresholds (figure 7). This observation is fundamentally similar across ages: we find no correlation between AI and age for verbal fluency, reading stories, auditory response naming, or listening to stories ($r^2 < 0.2$). Furthermore, variability seen in normal and patient populations suggests that language functions do not occur in anterior frontal or parietal areas. Non-dominant activation in homologous regions, present and similar across age groups, may assume capacity to sustain language functions resulting from left hemisphere insults. "Reorganization" appears to occur in homotopic right hemisphere and on the margins of traditional language areas in the dominant hemisphere (figure 8).

Functional MRI has also being increasingly used to examine neural networks implicated (or not) in developmental language disorders. Many of the early studies were conducted in adults, and now are being performed in children. Studies in patients with dyslexia show different activation patterns compared to normal controls for phonological processing tasks. For example, in one single word reading and matching task, dyslexic subjects exhibit greater activation in inferior frontal and right temporo-parietal regions and little activation in left temporal regions (Pugh, Mencl, Jenner et al. 2000). The patterns seen are also regionally restricted, rather than diffuse, and imply the use of an alternative, and perhaps less efficient or immature, strategy for reading processing (Pugh et al.1996; Pugh, Mencl, Shaywitz et al. 2000; Pugh, Mencl, Jenner et al. 2000; Dapretto et al. 1996). Furthermore, preliminary evidence suggests that intervention results in "normalization" of activation patterns for the task (Dapretto et al. 1996; Pugh, Mencl, Jenner et al. 2000).

CONCLUSION

Functional MRI provides a powerful means of studying the organization of cognitive functions in children during normal health and in disease. Current methods are restricted to children five years, perhaps four, and older. By this time language networks are firmly established. They are highly lateralized and regionally specific. For the most part they are fundamentally similar to those of adults. Differences likely represent different strategies that may be normal variant, immature, or pathological, but these too are regionally restricted. In patients with neurologic injury in early life, language networks remain confined to certain brain regions—dorsolateral prefrontal cortex (BA 44, 45, 47, 46, 6) and temporal, temporal parietal regions (21, 22, 37, 39) and may be left or right sided—but are never seen outside these areas in occipital, superior parietal, mesial, or anterior frontal regions. These findings suggest that the regions that can sustain language functions are regionally specific and evolutionarily selected. Evidence from the epilepsy and stroke population suggests that contra-lateral homologous brain regions and adjacent areas retain some capacity to sustain language function in the setting of injury, and that this capacity is retained in diminishing capacity through adolescence, and perhaps in a fortunate few, into later life.

ACKNOWLEDGMENTS

Supported by NINDS KO8 NS1663 (WDG), the Epilepsy Research Branch, NINDS, a Grant form the Board of Lady Visitors (WDG, LMB) and an American Epilepsy Society & Epilepsy Foundation of America Award (LMB).

REFERENCES

Ahmad, Z., Balsamo, L., Xu, B., Theodore, W. H., and Gaillard, W. D. 2001. Auditory Comprehension of Language in Young Children: Neural Networks Identified with fMRI. American Neurologic Association Meeting. Chicago.

Balsamo, L. M., Xu, B., Grandin, C. B., Petrella, J. R., Braniecki, S. H., Elliott, T. K., and Gaillard, W. D. 2002. Left hemisphere language dominance with an auditory naming naming task in children: An fMRI study. *Archives of Neurology* 59:1168–74.

Bates, E., Thal, D., Vicari, S., Trauner, D., Fenson, J., Aram, D., Eisele, J., and Nass, R. 1997. From first words to grammar in children with focal brain injury. In *Developmental Neuropsychology* 13:447–76.

Bates, E. 1999. Plasticity, localization and language development. In *The Changing Nervous System: Neurobehavioral Consequences of Early Brain Disorders*, eds. S. Broman and J. M. Fletcher. New York: Oxford University Press.

Bavelier, D., Corina, D., Jezzard, P., Padmanabhan, S., Clark, V. P., Karni, A., Prinster, A., Braun, A., Lalwani, A., Rauschecker, J. P., Turner, R., and Neviller, H. 1997. Sentence reading: A functional MRI study at 4 Tesla. *Journal of Cognitive Neuroscience* 9:664–86.

Benson, R. R., Fitzgerald, D. B., LeSueur, L. L., Kennedy, D. N., Kwong, K. K., Buchbinder, B. R., Davis, T. L., Weisskoff, R. M., Talavage, T. M., Logan, W. J., Cosgrove, G. R., Belliveau, J. W., and Rosen, B. R. 1999. Language dominance determined by whole brain functional MRI in patients with brain lesions. *Neurology* 52:798–809.

Billingsley, R. L., McAndrews, M. P., Crawley, A. P., and Mikulis, D. J. 2001. Functional MRI of phonological and semantic processing in temporal lobe epilepsy. *Brain* 124:1218–27.

Binder, J., Achten, R., Constable, T., Detre, J., Gaillard, W. D., Jack, C., and Loring, D. 2002. fMRI in epilepsy. *Epilepsia* (Suppl) 43:51–63.

Binder, J. R., Swanson, S. J., Hammeke, T. A., Morris, G. L., Mueller, W. M., Fischer, M., Benbadis, S., Frost, J. S., Rao, S. M., and Haughton, V. M. 1996. Determination of language dominance using functional MRI: A comparison with the Wada test. *Neurology* 46:978–84.

Bookheimer, S. Y., Zeffiro, T., Blaxton, T., Malow, B., Gaillard, W. D., Sato, S., Kufta, C., Fedio, P., and Theodore, W. H. 1997. A Direct Comparison of PET Activation and Electrocortical Stimulation Mapping for Language Localization. *Neurology* 48:1056–65.

Bookheimer, S. Y., Zeffiro, T. A., Blaxton, T. A., Gaillard, W. D., Malow, B., and Theodore, W. H. 1998. Regional cerebral blood flow during auditory responsive naming: Evidence for cross-modality neural activation. *NeuroReport* 9:2409–13.

Bookheimer, S. Y., Zeffiro, T. A., Blaxton, T. A., Gaillard, W. D., and Theodore, W. H. 2000. Activation of language cortex with automatic speech tasks. *Neurology* 55:1151–7.

Booth, J. R., MacWhinney, B., Thulborn, K. R., Sacco, K., Voyvodic, J., and Feldman, H. M. 1999. Functional organization of activation patterns in children: Whole brain fMRI imaging during three different cognitive tasks. *Progress in Neuropsychopharmacology Biological Psychiatry* 23:669–82.

Booth, J. R., MacWhinney, B., Thulborn, K. R., Sacco, K., Voyvodic, J. T., and Feldman, H. M. 2000. Developmental and lesion effects in brain activation during sentence comprehension and mental rotation. *Developmental Neuropsychology* 18:139–69.

Breier, J. I., Simos, P. G., Wheless, J. W., Constantinou, J. E., Baumgartner, J. E., Venkataraman, V., and Papanicolaou, A. C. 2001. Language dominance in children as determined by magnetic source imaging and the intracarotid amobarbital procedure: A comparison. *Journal of Child Neurology* 16:124–30.

Casey, B. J., Cohen, J. D., Jezzard, P., Turner, R., Noll, D. C., Trainor, R. J., Giedd, J., Kaysen, D., Hertz-Pannier, L., and Rapoport, J. L. 1995. Activation of prefrontal cortex in children during a nonspatial working memory task with functional MRI. *Neuroimage* 2:221–29.

Casey, B. J., Trainor, R. J., Orendi, J. L., Schubert, A. B., Nystrom, L. E., Giedd, J. N., Castellanos, F. X., Haxby, J. V., Noll, D. C., Cohen, J. D. et al. 1997. A developmental functional MRI study of prefrontal activation during performance of a Go-No-Go task. *Journal of Cognitive Neuroscience* 9:835–47.

Cohen, R. M., Gross, M., Semple, W. E., Nordahl, T. E., and Sunderland, T. 1994. The metabolic brain pattern of young subjects given scopolamine. *Experimental Brain Research* 100:133–43.

Dapretto, M., Bookheimer, S. Y., Cohen, M. S. et al. 1996. FMRI of language in dyslexic and normally developing children. *Neuroimage* 3:S434.

Dapretto, M., and Bookheimer, S. Y. 1999. Form and content: Dissociating syntax and semantics in sentence comprehension. *Neuron* 24:427–32.

Demb, J. B., Desmond, J. E., Wagner, A. D., Vaidya, C. J., Glover, G. H., and Gabrieli, J. D. E. 1995. Semantic encoding and retrieval in the left inferior and prefrontal cortex: A functional MRI study of task difficulty and process specificity. *Journal of Neuroscience* 15:5870–8.

Devinsky, O., Perrine, K., Llinas, R., Luciano, D. J., and Dogali, M. 1993. Anterior temporal language areas in patients with early onset temporal lobe epilepsy. *Annals of Neurology* 34:727–32.

Fernandez, G., de Greiff, A., von Oertzen, J., Reuber, M., Lun, S., Klaver, P., Ruhlmann, J., Reul, J., and Elger, C. E. 2001. Language mapping in less than 15 minutes: Real-time functional MRI during routine clinical investigation. *Neuroimage* 14:585–94.

Fitzgerald, D. B., Cosgrove, G. R., Ronner, S., Jiang, H., Buchbinder, B. R., Belliveau, J. W., Rosen, B. R., and Benson, R. R. 1997. Location of language in the cortex: A comparison between functional MR imaging and electro-cortical stimulation. *American Journal of NR* 18:1529–39.

Gaillard, W. D., Hertz-Pannier, L., Mott, S. H., Barnett, A. S., LeBihan, D., and Theodore, W. H. 2000a. Functional anatomy of cognitive development: fMRI of verbal fluency in children and adults. *Neurology* 54:180–85.

Gaillard, W. D., Bookheimer, S. Y., and Cohen, M. 2000b. The Use of fMRI in Neocortical Epilepsy. *Advances in Neurology Neocortical Epilepsy* 84:391–404.

Gaillard, W. D., Xu, B., Balsamo, L., Grandin, C. B., Papero, P., Weinstein, S., Conry, J., Pearl, P., Spanaki, M. V., Petrella, J. R., Sato, S., and Theodore, W. H. 2000c. fMRI. Identification of Language Dominance in Patients with Complex Partial Epilepsy using an Auditory Based Language Comprehension Task. American Epilepsy Society, Platform Presentation. *Epilepsia* 41 (Suppl 7):83.

Gaillard, W. D., and Theodore, W. H. 2000d. Mapping language in epilepsy with functional neuroimaging. *The Neuroscientist* 6:391–401.

Gaillard, W. D., Pugliese, M., Grandin, C. B., Braniecki, S. H., Kondapaneni, P., Hunter, K., Xu, B., Petrella, J. R., Balsamo, L., and Basso, G. 2001a. Cortical localization of reading in normal children: A fMRI language study. *Neurology* 57:47–54.

Gaillard, W. D., Grandin, C. B., and Xu, B. 2001b. Developmental Aspects of Pediatric fMRI: Considerations for Image Acquisition, Analysis, and Interpretation. *NeuroImage* 13:239–49.

Gaillard, W. D., Balsamo, L., Xu, B., Grandin, C. B., Braniecki, S. H., Papero, P., Weinstein, S., Conry, J., Pearl, P. L., Sato, S., Jabbari, B., Vezina, L. G., Frattali, C., and Theodore, W. H. 2002. Language dominance in partial epilepsy patients identified with an fMRI reading task. *Neurology* 59:256–65.

Harvey, A. S., Anderson, D., Jackson, G., Anderson, V., Saling, M., Abbott, D., Kean, M., and Wellard, M. 1999. Functional MRI lateralization of expressive language in children with partial epilepsy and left hemisphere lesions. *Epilepsia* 40 (Suppl7):183.

Hertz-Pannier, L., Gaillard, W. D., Mott, S. H., Cuenod, C. A., Bookheimer, S. Y., Weinstein, S., Conry, J., Papero, P. H., Schiff, S. J., Le Bihan, D., and Theodore, W. H. 1997. Noninvasive assessment of language dominance in children and adolescents with functional MRI: A preliminary study. *Neurology* 48:1003–12.

Holland, S. K., Plante, E., Weber Byars, A. et al. 2001. Normal fMRI brain activation patterns in children performing a verb generation task. *NeuroImage* 14:837–43.

Hunter, K. E., Blaxton, T. A., Bookheimer, S. Y., Figlozzi, C., Gaillard, W. D., Grandin, C., Anyanwu, A., and Theodore, W. H. 1999. (15) O water positron emission tomography in language localization: A study comparing positron emission tomography visual and computerized region of interest analysis with the WADA test. *Annals of Neurology* 45:662–65.

Just, M. A., Carpenter, P. A., Keller, T. A., Eddy, W. F., and Thulborn, K. R. 1996. Brain activation modulated by sentence comprehension. *Science* 274:114–16.

Keene, D. L., Logan, W. J., McAndrews, M. P., Crawley, A. P., and Mikulius, D. J. 2000. A comparison of three functional MRI language paradigms in children. *Epilepsia* 41(Suppl7):193.

Kurthen, M., Helmstaedter, C., Linke, D. B., Solymosi, L., Elger, C. E., and Schramm, J. 1992. Interhemispheric dissociation of expressive and receptive language functions in patients with complex-partial seizures: An amobarbital study. Department of Neurosurgery, University Hospital of Bonn, Germany. *Brain and Language* 43:694–712.

Lehéricy, S., Cohen, L., Bazin, B., Samson, S., Giacomini, E., Routgetet, R., Hertz-Pannier, L., LeBihan, D., Marsault, C., and Baulac, M. 2000. Functional MR evaluation of temporal and frontal language dominance compared with the Wada test. *Neurology* 54:1625–33.

Lenneberg, E. H. 1967. *Biological Foundations of Language.* New York: Wiley.

Lia, T., Guang, Chen, Z., Ostergaard, L., Hindmarsh, T., and Moseley, M. E. 2000. Quantification of cerebral blood flow by bolus tracking and artery spin tagging methods. *Magnetic Resonance Imaging* 18:503–12.

Logan, W. J. 1999. Functional magnetic resonance imaging in children. *Seminar of Pediatric Neurology* 6:78–86.

Logothetis, N. K., Pauls, J., Augath, M., Trinath, T., and Oeltermann, A. 2001. Neurophysiological investigation of the basis of the fMRI signal. *Nature* 412:150–57.

Loring, D. W., Strauss, E., Hermann, B. P., Perrine, K., Trenerry, M. R., Barr, W. B., Westerveld, M., Chelune, G. J., Lee, G. P., and Meador, K. J. 1999. Effects of anomalous language representation on neuropsychological performance in temporal lobe epilepsy. *Neurology* 53:260–64.

Malonek, D., Dirnagl, U., Lindauer, U., Yamada, K., Kanno, and I., Grinvald, A. 1997. Vascular imprints of neuronal activity: Relationships between the dynamics of cortical blood flow, oxygenation, and volume changes following sensory stimulation. *Proceedings of the National Academy of Science* 94:14826–31.

Mazoyer, B. M., Tzourio, N., Frak, V., Syrota, A., Murayama, N., Levrier, O., Salamon, G., Dehaene, S., Cohen, L., and Mehler, J. 1993. The cortical representation of speech. *Journal of Cognitive Neuroscience* 5:467–79.

Moonen, C. T. W., and Bandettini, P. A. 2000. *Functional MRI.* Springer: New York.

Müller, R. A., Behen, M. E., Rothermel, R. D., Muzik, O., Chakraborty, P. K., and Chugani, H. T. 1999. Brain organization for language in children, adolescents, and adults with left hemisphere lesion: A PET study. *Progress in NeuroPsychopharmacological and Biological Psychiatry* 23:657–68.

Nelson, C. A., Monk, C. S., Lin, J., Carver, L. J., Thomas, K. M., and Truwit, C. L. 2000. Functional neuroanatomy of spatial working memory in children. *Developmental Psychology* 36:109–16.

Ojemann, G. A., Ojemann, J., Lettich, E., and Berger, M. 1989. Cortical language localization in left, dominant hemisphere: An electrical stimulation mapping investigation in 117 patients. *Journal of Neurosurgery* 71: 316–26.

Pardo, J. V., and Fox, P. T. 1993. Preoperative assessment of the cerebral hemispheric dominance for language with CBF PET. *Human Brain Mapping* 1:57–68.

Poldrack, R. A., Wagner, A. D., Prull, M. W., Desmond, J. E., Glover, G. H., and Gabrieli, J. D. E. 1999. Functional specialization for semantic and phonological processing in the left inferior prefrontal cortex. *Neuroimage* 10:15–35.

Pugh, K. R., Shaywitz, B. A., Shaywitz, S. E., Constable, R. T., Skudlarski, P., Fulbright, R. K., Bronen, R. A., Shankweiler, D. P., Katz, L., Fletcher, J. M., and Gore, J. C. 1996. Cerebral organization of component processes in reading. *Brain* 119:1221–38.

Pugh, K. R., Mencl, W. E., Shaywitz, B. A., Shaywitz, S. E., Fulbright, R. K., Constable, R. T., Skudlarski, P., Marchione, K. E., Jenner, A. R.., Fletcher, J. M., Liberman, A. M., Shankweiler, D. P., Katz, L., Lacadie, C., and Gore, J. C. 2000. The angular gyrus in developmental dyslexia: task-specific differences in functional connectivity within posterior cortex. *Psychological Science* 11:51–56.

Pugh, K. R., Mencl, W. E., Jenner, A. R., Katz, L., Frost, S. J., Lee, J. R., Shaywitz, S. E., and Shaywitz, B. A. 2000. Functional neuroimaging studies of reading and reading disability (developmental dyslexia). *Mental Retardation and Developmental Disabilities Research Review* 6:207–13.

Pugliese, M., Gaillard, W. D, Basso, G., Braniecki, S. H., Xu, B., Balsamo, L. M., Nichelli, P., Cavazzuti, G. B., Grafman, J., and Theodore, W. H. 1999. Functional brain mapping of visual mental imagery in children. *Neuroimage* 9:S352.

Pujol, J., Deus, J., Losilla, J. M., and Capdevila, A. 1999. Cerebral lateralization of language in normal left-handed people studied by functional MRI. *Neurology* 52:1038–43.

Rasmussen, T., and Milner, B. 1977. The role of early left-brain injury in determining lateralization of cerebral speech functions. *Annals of New York Academy of Science* 229:335–69.

Schlagger, B. L., Brown, T. T., Lugar, H. M., Visscher, K. M., Miezin, F. M., and Petersen, S. E. 2002. Functional neuroanatomical differences between adults and school-age children in the processing of single words. *Science* 296: 1476–79.

Schlosser, M. J., Aoyagi, N., Fulbright, R. K., Gore, J. C., and McCarthy, G. 1998. Functional MRI studies of auditory comprehension. *Human Brain Mapping* 6:1–13.

Serafini, S., Steury, K., Richards, T., Corina, D., Abbott, R., Dager, S. R., and Berninger, V. 2001. Comparison of fMRI and PEPSI during language processing in children. *Magnetic Resonance Medicine* 45:217–25.

Springer, J. A., Binder, J. R., Hammeke, T. A., Swanson, S. J., Frost, J. A., Bellgowan, P. S., Brewer, C. C., Perry, H. M., Morris, G. L., and Mueller, W. M. 1999. Language dominance in neurologically normal and epilepsy subjects: A functional MRI study. *Brain* 122:2033–46.

Stapleton, S. R., Kiriakipoulos, E., Mikulis, D., Drake, J. M., Hoffman, H. J., Humphreys, R., Hwang, P, Otsubo, H., Holowka, S., Logan, W., and Rutka, J. T. 1997. Combined utility of functional MRI, cortical mapping, and frameless stereotaxy in the resection of lesions in eloquent areas of brain in children. *Pediatric Neurosurgery* 26:68–82.

Staudt, M., Pieper, T., Grodd, W., Winkler, P., Holthausen, H., and Krageloh-Mann, I. 2001. Functional MRI in a 6-year-old boy with unilateral cortical malformation: concordant representation of both hands in the unaffected hemisphere. *Neuropediatrics* 32:159–61.

Thomas, K. M., King, S. W., Franzen, P. L., Welsh, T. F., Berkowitz, A. L., Noll, D. C., Birmaher, V., Casey, B. J. 1999. A developmental functional MRI study of spatial working memory. *Neuroimage* 10:327–38.

Thomas, K. M., Drevets, W. C., Dahl, R. E., Ryan, N. D., Birmaher, B., Eccard, C. H., Axelson, D., Whalen, P. J., and Casey, B. J. 2001. Amygdala response to fearful faces in anxious and depressed children. *Archives of General Psychiatry* 58:1057–63.

Thompson-Schill, S. L., D'Esposito, M., Aguirre, G. K., and Farah, M. J. 1997. Role of left inferior prefrontal cortex in retrieval of semantic knowledge: A reevaluation. *Proceedings of the National Academy of Science USA* 23:14792–7.

Ulualp, S. O., Biswal, B. B., Yetkin, Z., and Kidder, T. M. 1998. Functional magnetic resonance imaging of auditory cortex in children. *The Laryngoscope* 108:1782–6.

Vaidya, C. J., Austin, G., Kirkorian, G., Ridlehuber, H. W., Desmond, J. E., Glover, G. H., and Gabrieli, J. D. 1998. Selective effects of methylphenidate in attention deficit hyperactivity disorder: A functional magnetic resonance study. *Proceedings of the National Academy of Science USA* 24:14494–9.

Woods, R. P., Dodrill, C. B., and Ojemann, G. A. 1988. Brain injury, handedness, and speech lateralization in a series of amobarbital studies. *Annals of Neurology* 23:510–18.

Ye, F. Q., Smith, A. M., Mattay, V. S., Ruttimann, U. E., Frank, J. A., Weinberger, D. R., and McLaughlin, A. C. 1998. Quantitation of regional cerebral blood flow increases in prefrontal cortex during a working memory task: A steady-state arterial spin-tagging study. *Neuroimage* 8:44–9.

Yetkin, F. Z., Swanson, S., Fischer, M., Akansel, G., Morris, G., Muller, W. et al. 1998. Functional MR of frontal lobe activation: Comparison with Wada language results. *American Journal of Neuroradiology* 19:1095–8.

Part • IV

Treatment and Outcome

Chapter • 9

Treatment of Primary Language Disorders in Early Childhood:
Evidence of Efficacy

Paul J. Yoder and Andrea S. McDuffie

There is a group of children who have delayed or disordered spoken language that cannot be explained by intellectual disabilities or sensory impairments (American Psychiatric Association 2000). Some have called this type of disorder primary language disorder (PLD), (Conti-Ramsden and Botting 2000). The motivation for identifying such children is based on an assumption that language therapy is effective and that early identification may lead to ameliorating the disorder. We conducted a review of the language intervention literature to determine the extent to which we have evidence that language therapy facilitates the language development of preschoolers with primary language disorder. A secondary interest was in identifying aspects of treatments and outcome measures that are associated with treatment effects.

The review included only internally valid language intervention studies on preschoolers or toddlers with primary language disorder. By targeting preschoolers and toddlers, we focused on a period considered by some to be a sensitive period for language intervention (Lieberman 1993). Others have argued that it is important to provide treatment during this period to prevent secondary and cumulative impairments (Hart and Risley 1995). By focusing on children with a particular disorder type (i.e., primary language disorder), the clinical population to which the review refers is well defined. By looking exclusively at studies with high internal validity (i.e., those that control for maturation and history as alternative explanations to the results), we can be more confident of the conclusions we draw.

This type of review is called a best evidence review (Slavin 1986). Slavin considered a best evidence review to be a rigorous, balanced review of only internally valid studies that are relevant to the review's motivating research question. Effect size information is used only for randomized group experiments, but other information is garnered across all internally valid research designs (e.g., presence or absence of strong evidence of a treatment effect). In our best evidence review, it is acknowledged that different research methods require different criteria for determining the presence of a treatment effect.

Best evidence reviews differ from traditional narrative reviews and meta-analyses on several points. First, traditional narrative reviews have less structure than best evidence reviews and thereby allow more avenues for influencing the outcome of the review (Slavin 1986). Meta-analyses (Lipsey and Wilson 2001) exclude studies that do not have the necessary information to compute effect size. For example, meta-analyses exclude single-subject designs and designs that compare treatments (Lipsey and Wilson 2001).

There have been several other recent reviews of the language intervention literature on children with PLD (Fey, in press; Fey and Proctor-Williams 2000; Law et. al. 1998; Leonard 1998; Weismer 2000). However, these have differed from the current review in the following ways. First, three have not covered all major aspects of language (e.g., grammar, semantics, pragmatics, and phonology) (Fey in press; Fey and Proctor-Williams 2000; Weismer 2000). Second, all five previous reviews have included data on older children as well as preschoolers and toddlers. Third, all five previous reviews have included data from studies with compromised internal validity (e.g., matched group designs or pre-experimental designs). Fourth, one review includes only studies that allow computation of effect sizes (Law et. al. 1998). Fifth, none of the five previous reviews has made a distinction concerning the degree to which the obtained effects indicate relatively trivial changes in language performance. Finally, four reviews did not include a systematic analysis of correlates of treatment effects (e.g., treatment effects might be stronger for vocabulary than for grammar) (Fey in press; Fey and Proctor-Williams 2000; Leonard 1998; Weismer 2000).

ASPECTS OF TREATMENT THAT MAY COVARY WITH TREATMENT EFFECTS

We set out to examine whether four aspects of treatment are associated with treatment effects: (a) amount of treatment, (b) specificity of

language goal, (c) treatment orientation, and (d) type of linguistic consequence to child communication. One might expect those studies
with more treatment to have stronger treatment effects than those
with less treatment. Recent speculation about the relative efficacy of
vocabulary intervention suggests that selecting specific target words is
more effective than targeting broader classes of vocabulary
(Girolametto, Pearce, and Weitzman 1996b). Child-oriented approaches (i.e., those that follow the child's attentional lead to select
materials and determine when to teach within the session) may be
more effective in facilitating generalized grammatical target use than
adult-oriented approaches (i.e.., those in which the adult controls materials and timing of teaching episodes) (Camarata, Nelson, and
Camarata 1994). Theory (Nelson 1989) and empirical work (Camarata,
Nelson, and Camarata 1994) suggest that treatments that use consequences such as expansions or recasts are likely to be more effective
than those that do not. When there has been research on these questions, there is usually only a single study in a single area of language
development. We do not know the extent to which these findings
replicate or generalize across aspects of language.

ASPECTS OF THE DEPENDENT VARIABLE THAT MAY COVARY WITH TREATMENT EFFECTS

We planned to test if the effect size or presence of a treatment effect
varied with the type of dependent variable measured. One way to cat-
egorize language outcomes is according to the level of evidence they
provide that the change in language performance is evidence of new
language ability (i.e., language development). Three such classes are
(a) associative learning/therapy set, (b) conceptual reorganization,
and (c) generalization to conversation.

Treatment effects on associative learning or therapy sets are considered weak evidence of an effect on language development by most
current language researchers (McCormick and Schiefelbusch 1990). If
the changes in a child's language performance can be explained by the
child simply learning the expectations of the therapist and using existing skills to fulfill these expectations, little has been gained. Effects on
spontaneous use of the language target in the treatment session may
be an example of this type of outcome. Additionally, if the child
makes a restricted association between a particular word and a particular referent, instead of learning that the word represents a category of referents, it will probably not be beneficial to the child outside
of the treatment session. Treatment effects on fast mapping of a nonsense word onto a single invented referent is an example of this type

of outcome. The key points here are that the outcome is measured only in the treatment session (no stimulus generalizaton has occurred) or in a way that allows a simple association to explain increased performance (no response generalization has occurred).

Two other classes of language outcomes (conceptual reorganization and generalization to conversation) represent stronger evidence of language development than does associative learning or therapy set outcomes (McCormick and Schiefelbusch 1990). When a child uses a new word for an unfamiliar exemplar of a trained category or uses a grammatical rule to generate a phrase for an unfamiliar exemplar of the rule, we have evidence of new conceptual or grammatical knowledge (Kamhi 1988). Structuralists call this type of learning conceptual reorganization (Kamhi 1988). When a child uses new language skills with someone other than the interventionist and this adult is also using a conversational style that is unlike the one used in treatment sessions, we are more confident that the child's new skills are likely to be used in the natural environment. We will call this class of effects evidence of generalization to conversations (Warren 1988).

Five other attributes of the language outcome were examined as potential covariates of treatment effects: (a) aspect of language, (b) degree to which the language target is measured, (c) modality of the outcome measure (i.e., production versus comprehension), (d) immediacy of the outcome measurement after the treatment phase, and (e) degree to which degree of language delay or deviance is measured. Some authors expect treatment effects on vocabulary to be stronger than effects on certain aspects of grammar (Pinker 1994). Treatment effects might be stronger for dependent variables that are closely matched to the language target. Production measures may reveal treatment effects more readily than comprehension measures because the former is a more direct measure of language. Comprehension measures require that we infer from the children's nonverbal behavior that they understand language (Tomasello and Mervis 1994). Dependent variables measured immediately after the end of treatment may be more likely to show treatment effects than measures taken several months or years after the end of treatment because multiple influences on individual differences on development can increase variance within experimental and control groups. Finally, treatment effects may vary by whether the dependent variable is a measure of degree of delay (i.e., standard scores) or level of skill development (i.e., raw scores or age equivalency scores). One might expect larger treatment effects or a higher probability of a treatment effect for dependent variables that reflect level of skill development than for variables reflecting degree of delay.

In summary, we used a best evidence method to guide our review of the language intervention literature. This involved identifying the most internally valid studies that tested the efficacy of language intervention on the language development of preschoolers and toddlers with primary language disorder. We then tested whether various aspects of the treatment methods and dependent variables accounted for variance in the probability of a treatment effect and in the magnitude of the effect sizes.

METHODS

Inclusion Criteria

Relevance criteria. For the study to be considered relevant to our research question, (a) some aspect of language had to be measured as a dependent variable, (b) at least one session in which therapeutic methods designed to facilitate grammatical, semantic, or pragmatic development had to be used, and (c) several population criteria had to be met. For single-subject studies, we considered only the results of participants that met our population criteria and at least two participants had to meet the criteria for a study to be included. For group designs to be included in our review, we required that 75% of the sample meet our criteria.

The relevant population was specified through criteria for chronological age, expressive language delay or disorder, nonverbal intelligence, and hearing ability. We included children under 61 months of age. The general description of the selection criteria for primary language disorder (PLD) was (a) substantial expressive language delay/disorder, (b) nonverbal intelligence above the range associated with intellectual disabilities, (c) hearing within normal limits. We included both expressive language disorders and mixed receptive-expressive disorders (American Psychiatric Association 2000). We recognized that these criteria could possibly result in inclusion of some studies with participants that did not fit the strict definition of specific language impairment (Stark and Tallal 1981).

To define expressive language delay, we set the criterion level of delay at or below the 10th percentile (i.e., 1.2 *SD* below the mean) on at least one norm-referenced expressive language test, excluding phonology tests. We anticipated that older studies would report only age equivalency scores. In such cases, we included the study when 75% of the sample had developmental quotients (age equivalent/chronological age) of .70 or greater on at least one expressive language test. We selected this developmental quotient because it was the lowest developmental quotient that corresponded with the 10th percentile on two standardized expressive language tests that also provided percentile rankings at 18 and 60 months: the Reynell Developmental

Language Scales (Reynell and Gruber 1990) and the Expressive One
Word Picture Vocabulary Test (Gardner 1990).

The inclusion criterion for nonverbal intelligence was a standard
score of 75 or above. We anticipated that many of the studies would
not administer a nonverbal intelligence test. In such cases, scores at or
above 75 on an intelligence test that included verbally loaded items
met the criterion. The rationale for this decision was that most language delayed children score lower on intelligence tests with verbally
loaded items than on intelligence tests with low or no verbal loading.
Therefore, children that scored in the non-retarded range on verbally
loaded tests were highly likely to score in this range on nonverbal intelligence tests. We also anticipated that several of the studies would
not administer any intelligence test. Two methods were used in such
cases. First, if the study authors indicated that no concern or evidence
of mental retardation was present, the intelligence criterion was met.
Second, if scores on all receptive language tests that were administered exceeded a standard score of 74, the intelligence criterion was
met. The rationale for the latter decision was that it is unusual for receptive language level to exceed nonverbal intelligence level (Miller
1999). Therefore, if the receptive language level was above our criterion level, there is a high probability that nonverbal intelligence was
as well. Finally, it was anticipated that some studies that did not include intelligence tests or that report no concern of mental retardation,
would use receptive tests that only reported age equivalent scores. In
such cases, studies were included if they had receptive developmental
quotients of .80 or above. This criterion developmental quotient was
selected because it was the highest derived from conversion charts for
18 and 60 months on the Reynell Developmental Language Scales
(Reynell and Gruber 1990) and for 30 and 60 months on the Peabody
Picture Vocabulary Test III (Dunn and Dunn 1997).

To pass our hearing criteria, studies had to indicate that there
was no evidence of hearing impairment. This could be accomplished
by indicating that participants had passed a hearing screening or if authors reported no concern or evidence of hearing impairment.

Internal validity criteria. Our internal validity criteria were
based on research designs that controlled for maturation and history
as threats to internal validity. These were: (a) randomized between-
group experiments; (b) within-subject randomized group experiments; (c) pre-post designs with nonsense or very unfamiliar targets
(i.e., those that are highly unlikely to be learned outside of the experimental treatment); or (d) single-subject designs that controlled for
maturation and history and are appropriate for addressing effects on
development. Single-subject designs that were judged to control for

maturation and history were: (a) certain types of multiple baseline across subjects and targets; and (b) adapted alternating treatment designs with equivalent but different language goals. Multiple baseline designs that were accepted were those that: (a) showed change in slope or level of the dependent variable in the treatment phase that could not be explained by continuation of baseline data slope; (b) showed less than 10% of treatment phase data that overlapped with baseline data; and (c) showed a change in the slope or level of the dependent variable within one month after the onset of treatment. The adapted alternating treatment studies that were accepted were those whose investigators created a pool of equally learnable, but different, language targets (e.g., vocabulary words) that were randomly assigned to treatment conditions. Reversal designs (i.e., designs in which the dependent variable was expected, and did, return to baseline when the treatment was withdrawn) were not included because measures of language development should not return to baseline after treatment is withdrawn.

The Review Process

The articles for review were selected by three methods. First, we conducted a computer-aided literature review using *PsychInfo* and *Medline*. The descriptors used were: *language and (impair* or disorder*) and (child* or toddler* or preschooler*) and (intervention or treatment or therapy)*. Second, we identified articles that were judged to have high internal validity by a recent meta-analysis on language intervention for children with primary disorders in language (Law et al. 1998). Third, we identified articles from the reference sections of four reviews of language intervention in children with language disorders (Fey in press; Fey and Proctor-Williams 2000; Leonard 1998; Weismer 2000). Fourth, we identified articles cited in the identified intervention studies that we had not previously identified.

Procedures

After identifying the appropriate articles, the following aspects of each were summarized for all articles, regardless of research design: (a) research design, (b) sample size, (c) sample description, (d) aspect of language measured as outcome, (e) presence/absence of maintenance check (if present, duration of interval to maintenance check), (f) amount of treatment, (g) specificity of language goal, (h) interventionist, and (i) aspect of language targeted. Two other aspects of the treatment that were specified were: (a) if child's attentional lead was followed to determine the timing and content of teaching episodes, and (b) which consequent events to child communication were used (if any). When the treatment description indicated that the treatment followed the child's attentional lead, the treatment was considered child oriented. Otherwise, the treatment was considered adult oriented.

For studies using group designs, we recorded 6 aspects of the dependent variable. First, we indicated the degree of match between the outcome and the language target (i.e., no target, same aspect and same level of specificity, same aspect but broader level of specificity, different aspect of language than target). Second, we recorded whether the outcome was a standard score or percentile ranking (a measure of degree of delay) versus a raw score or age equivalent (a measure of skill level). Third, we indicated whether the examiner or informant was also the child's interventionist. Fourth, we recorded whether the examiner used an interaction style during the assessment procedure that was not used in the treatment sessions. Fifth, we indicated whether generalization across exemplars/sentence stems was tested, we recorded whether a standardized language test or language sample was used as the dependent variable's measurement context.

For studies using a single-subject design, we summarized four aspects of dependent variables. First, we indicated whether the dependent variable was measured within the treatment session. Second, we indicated whether the dependent variable was measured using the same materials used in the treatment sessions. Third, we indicated what, if any, type of generalization was tested (i.e., across persons, across materials, across sentence stems, across interaction styles, across locations). For within-treatment session and generalization measures, we indicated the proportion of subjects with strong evidence that the treatment caused the changes in the dependent variable. The criteria used to determine strong evidence of a treatment effect are given below.

From the description of the dependent variables, the first or second author who summarized the article classified the dependent variable into one of the three types of evidence of language development. The dependent variable was classified as associative learning or therapy set performance if one of these three criteria were met. First, the interventionist was the adult who was interacting with the child when the dependent variable was measured. Second, the adult interacting with the child was using an interaction style similar to that used in treatment sessions. Or third, the referent for the target word or phrase was the same as that used during the treatment sessions. The dependent variable was classified as evidence of conceptual reorganization if one of the following criteria were met: (a) generalization to non-trained exemplars or sentence stems was shown, and (b) standardized tests were used as the measurement instrument. The latter was considered acceptable because it was improbable that training exemplars and sentence stems were those used in standardized test items. The dependent variable was classified as evidence of generalization to conversation if all three of the following criteria were met: (a) the child used the target with an adult other than the interventionist, (b) the examiner's interaction style was different from the style used during treatment, and (c) the measurement context was a conversational language sample.

The evidence used to infer strong evidence of a treatment effect varied by research design. Statistically significant differences between experimental and control groups on the post-treatment or follow-up measures was evidence of a treatment effect in studies using a randomized between-group experiment. Statistically significant differences between conditions was evidence of a treatment effect in studies using a randomized within-subject group experiment. Statistically significant differences between obtained scores and chance was evidence of a treatment effect in studies using a pre-post nonsense target design. Strong evidence of a treatment effect in multiple baseline design studies was present when several conditions existed: (a) effects replicated across participants or targets (i.e., in more than two participants), (b) changes in slope or level of the dependent variable occurred within one month after the onset of the treatment phase, (c) the slope of the baseline trend line was flat or descending, and (d) less than 10% of the treatment phase data overlapped with the highest baseline data point. Strong evidence of a treatment effect in adapted alternating treatment designs was clear separation of the slope of growth trends for at least two subjects.

For randomized between-group experiments, we computed the standardized mean difference between post-treatment scores adjusted for sample size (Lipsey and Wilson 2001). The standardized mean difference needs to be adjusted for sample size because Hedges (1981) found that standardized mean differences are upwardly biased when based on small samples, particularly samples less than 20. When means and standard deviations were not available in the article, we estimated the standardized mean difference from the p value and sample sizes (Lipsey and Wilson 2001). It should be noted that pre-post effect sizes in pre-post designs using nonsense targets do not mean the same as the standardized mean differences between groups (Lipsey and Wilson 2001). The latter is more widely used and most generally understood. Therefore, the former will not be analyzed or discussed here.

Levels of Analysis Used

One can summarize and analyze literature review results at the study level or at the dependent variable level. When summarized at the dependent variable level, we summarize across studies. That is, each test of a treatment effect is considered a separate and equally weighted piece of information, regardless of how many dependent variables are tested in a given study. When summarized at the study level, we compute the probability of a treatment effect for each study by dividing the number of tests for treatment effects that showed strong evidence of an effect by the total number of tests. For randomized between-group experiments, we compute the average effect sizes across all dependent variables in the study (Lipsey and Wilson 2001).

For research design and treatment description variables, we described the review results by study. The information at the study level weighs each study equally. This is appropriate for thinking about the type of studies included in the review. For description of the dependent variables, we described the review results at the dependent variable level. The dependent variable level of analysis is the most common type used in literature reviews in speech-language pathology. However, such a method gives more weight to studies that test multiple dependent variables.

When identifying the correlates of effect size or presence and probability of a treatment effect, one can also analyze the results at the study level and at the dependent variable level. Analyses at the study level meet the assumptions of commonly used (i.e., asymptotic) statistical tests better than do analyses at the dependent variable level. The statistical assumption usually violated by dependent variable level analyses is called sampling independence, which refers to the assumption that analysis units do not influence each other (Hayes 1996). The analysis unit for study level analyses is the study. The analysis unit for dependent variable level analyses is the dependent variable.

One reason most review authors analyze their results at the level of the dependent variable is that there are many more dependent variables across studies than there are studies. Treating each dependent variable as a separate unit of analysis increases the statistical power over analyses that treat studies as the separate unit of analysis. However, analyzing the dependent variable as a separate unit of analysis is a violation of the assumption of sampling independence because many dependent variables come from the same sample and are treated with the same intervention method. The possible problem is that when we violate the assumption of independent sampling units, there may be elevated type I error rates (Hayes 1996).

We addressed this issue in two ways. First, where feasible, we examined correlates of effect sizes and probability of a treatment effect at the study level. We tested whether research design and treatment type were correlates of treatment effects. Second, when testing whether treatment effects varied by attributes of the dependent variable (i.e., a variable that could not be analyzed at the study level without losing much information), we analyzed at the dependent variable level and used permutation tests (Good 2000). Many researchers implicitly or explicitly claim permutation tests are less affected by violations of the assumption of independent sampling units than are asymptotic tests by using the former method to analyze single-subject data (Edgington 1984; Ferron and Onghena 1996; Levin, Marascuilo, and Hubert 1978).

RESULTS

Fifty-seven articles were reviewed for the inclusion criteria. Thirty-six articles were rejected for reasons summarized in table I. Appendix A identifies the rejected studies and displays the reasons for rejection by study. The most frequent reasons for rejection were that the children were over 60 months of age and/or the study had inadequate internal validity. Insufficient expressive language delay was a close second, followed by unclear or inadequate cognitive level. One study was excluded due to inclusion of participants with evidence of hearing impairment.

Twenty-one articles fit all of the inclusion criteria. These described 23 different studies, each of which were judged to describe separate and unique samples of participants.

Description of the Included Studies

Research designs represented. Forty-three percent (i.e., ten) of the studies were randomized between group designs (Fey et al. 1993; Wilcox and Leonard 1978; Gibbard 1994, experiments 1 and 2;

Table I.   Summary of the reasons studies were rejected (n = 36).

Reasons for rejecting	Number of studies rejected for this reason*
At least 25% of sample was over 60 months	12
Inadequate internal validity	12
At least 25% of sample had expressive levels higher than the 10th percentile or such information was missing	11
At least 25% of sample had evidence of non-normal IQs or such information was missing	6
Sample included children with diagnosed hearing loss	1

*Total exceeds 36 due to multiple reasons for exclusion for some studies.

Robertson and Weismer 1997 study 1, 1999; Girolametto, Pearce, and Weitzman 1996b, 1997; Rice, Buhr, and Nemeth 1990; Whitehurst et al. 1989). Twenty-two percent (i.e., five) were pre-post designs with nonsense targets (Schwartz et al. 1987; Schwartz 1988; Swisher et al. 1995; Swisher and Snow 1994) or very unfamiliar targets (Leonard et al. 1982). Four (17%) were multiple baselines (Hedge and Gierut 1979; Connell 1986a; Olswang and Coggins 1984; Robertson and Weismer 1997, study 2). Two (.09%) were adapted alternating treatment designs (Olswang et al. 1986; Weismer, Murray-Branch, and Miller 1993). Two (.09%) were within-subject group experiments (Camarata, Nelson, and Camarata 1994; Connell and Stone 1992).

Characteristics of the Treatments Represented. We could estimate the average number of therapy hours each participant received in all but two studies (Whitehurst et al. 1989; Wilcox and Leonard 1978). Over the remaining 21 studies, the grand average (average of the study averages) for the number of hours of therapy time was 16 hours ($SD = 16$; min = 1; max = 59; two studies lacked this information). The two studies with an average of one hour of therapy time were fast mapping studies (Robertson and Weismer 1997, experiments 1 and 2).

We could not determine specific language targets for six studies (Gibbard 1994, experiments 1 and 2; Robertson and Weismer 1997, experiments 1 and 2, 1999; Whitehurst et al. 1989). In 74% (17) of the studies, the authors stated that specific words, specific grammatical structures, or specific semantic relations were goals of the intervention. Of these 17, 47% (i.e., eight) targeted specific vocabulary words (Girolametto, Pearce, and Weitzman 1996b, 1997; Olswang et al. 1986; Rice, Buhr, and Nemeth 1990; Weismer, Murray-Branch, and Miller 1993; Leonard et al. 1982; Schwartz et al. 1987; Schwartz 1988), 41% (seven) targeted specific grammatical structures (Camarata, Nelson, and Camarata 1994; Fey et al. 1993; Hedge and Gierut 1979; Wilcox and Leonard 1978; Connell and Stone 1992; Swisher et al. 1995; Swisher and Snow 1994), and 12% (two) targeted specific semantic relations (Connell 1986a; Olswang and Coggins 1984).

We could judge whether the study used a child oriented versus an adult oriented treatment approach in all but 3 studies (Gibbard 1994, experiment 1 and 2; Olswang and Coggins 1984). In the remaining 20 studies, exactly half were adult oriented (Connell and Stone 1992; Swisher et al. 1995; Swisher and Snow 1994;Wilcox and Leonard 1978; Hedge and Gierut 1979; Connell 1986a; Olswang et al. 1986; Weismer, Murray-Branch, and Miller 1993; Rice, Buhr, and Nemeth 1990; Schwartz et al. 1987) and half were child oriented or hybrid (Camarata, Nelson, and Camarata 1994; Fey et al. 1993; Schwartz 1988;

Whitehurst et al. 1989; Robertson and Weismer 1999; Robertson and Weismer 1997, studies 1 and 2; Girolametto, Pearce, and Weitzman 1996b, 1997; Leonard et al. 1982).

We could judge whether the study used a treatment with consequences to child communication that added linguistic information to the child's platform utterance in all but three studies (Gibbard 1994, studies 1 and 2; Olswang and Coggins 1984). Of these 20 studies, 40% (eight) used treatments in which the interventionist used consequences to child utterances that added linguistic information to the child's preceding platform utterance (e.g., linguistic mapping, expansions, recasts) (Swisher et al. 1995; Swisher and Snow 1994; Weismer, Murray-Branch, and Miller 1993; Fey et al. 1993; Camarata, Nelson, and Camarata 1994; Whitehurst et al. 1989; Robertson and Weismer 1999; Girolametto, Pearce, and Weitzman 1996a). The remaining 60% (12) used consequences that did not add linguistic information (e.g., praise, corrective feedback) or did not use consequences.

Characteristics of the language dependent variables. Because most studies had more than one dependent variable, these data are presented at the dependent variable level. Across studies, treatment effects were tested on 107 language outcome variables. Table II indicates the characteristics of the dependent variables. It should be noted that most of the dependent variables constituted the weakest evidence of language development (i.e., associative learning/therapy set). However, a large (47%) minority represented the two stronger types of evidence of language development: conceptual reorganization and generalization to conversations. Most of these (62%) variables (31/50) tested for evidence of conceptual reorganization. It should also be noted that 74% of the dependent variables were measures of vocabulary (40% of 107) or grammar (34%). Eighty-nine percent of the dependent variables were measures of production. Finally, of the dependent variables in the 17 studies that had specific language targets (66% of the dependent variables), 59% (39) of these outcomes were measured at a specific level and were measuring the same aspect of language that was targeted in treatment. In addition, 21% (14) were measures of a nontargeted aspect of language, and 20% (13) of the outcomes were general measures of the targeted aspect of language.

Surprisingly, only two (2%) of the dependent variables were measures of degree of delay (i.e., standard scores) and these were from the same study (Whitehurst et. al. 1989). Only two of the dependent variables tested maintenance of gains (2%) and they were from the same study (Robertson and Weismer 1997, study 1). Additionally, the length of interval between the end of the treatment phase and the maintenance assessment was only 3 weeks.

Table II.   Characteristics of the dependent variables (DVs).

Characteristics of DVs	Proportion out 107 DVs	# of DVs
Evidence of language development		
Associative learning/therapy set	.53	57
Conceptual reorganization	.30	31
Generalization to conversation	.18	19
Aspect of language measured		
Vocabulary	.40	43
Grammar	.34	36
Phonology	.09	10
Talkativeness	.07	7
Global	.06	6
Semantic relations	.04	4
Modality		
Production	.89	95
Comprehension	.11	12
Specificity and aspect of DV visa vie target		
Nonspecific target	.38	41
Same aspect as target; specific level of measurement	.36	39
Different aspect than target	.13	14
Same aspect as target; general level of measurement	.12	13

Summary of the Treatment Effects

At the study level, the average probability of strong evidence of a treatment effect was 51% (SD = .41%). In the randomized between-group experiments (10 studies), the grand average of the adjusted effect sizes (i.e., average of the average adjusted effect size) was 1.22 (SD = .71). This average is significantly different from zero (t = 5.37; $p < .001$). At the dependent variable level, strong evidence of a treatment effect was found in 56% of the 107 outcomes tested. Of the randomized between-group experiments, there were 75 effects tested. The average adjusted effect size was 1.07 (SD = .62).

Correlates of Treatment Effects

Does the probability of a treatment effect vary by research design?   The average probability of strong evidence of a treatment effect did vary by research design (F = 9.01; p = .002; eta squared = .50; observed power = .95). The average probability of strong evidence of a treatment effect was .79 (SD = .26) for randomized between-group experiments, .30 (SD = .45) for pre-post nonsense/unfamiliar word designs, and .14 (SD = .27) for single-subject designs. An insufficient number (i.e., two) of studies used within-subject group experimental designs to warrant inclusion in this analysis.

Does the probability of a treatment effect or average effect size vary by characteristics of the treatment? The probability of strong evidence of a treatment effect did not vary by average amount of treatment ($r = .25$; $p = .28$; observed power $= .20$), or differ by specificity of language target ($F = 2.33$; $p = .14$; eta squared $= .10$; observed power $= .31$) or presence of consequences that provided linguistic information ($F = 1.38$; $p = .26$; eta squared $= .07$; observed power $= .20$). The low observed power is noteworthy and demonstrates why reviews tend to analyze at the dependent variable level.

The probability of strong evidence of a treatment effect did vary by treatment orientation ($F = 5.24$; $p = .03$; eta squared $= .23$; observed power $= .58$). The average probability of strong evidence of a treatment effect was .71 ($SD = .40$) for child oriented and hybrid treatments and .33 ($SD = .35$) for adult oriented treatments. The tests to examine potential covariates of average effect size at the study level were conducted on the ten randomized between-group experiments. The observed power for these analyses ranged from .06 to .16. The eta squares varied from .008 for specificity of language target to .21 for treatment orientation. None of the associations between characteristics of treatment and effect size were statistically significant. Again, the low observed power is noteworthy.

Does the probability of strong evidence for a treatment effect and adjusted effect size vary by characteristics of the dependent variable? We could only test the question for the types of evidence of language development, aspect of language, specificity and aspect match with language target, and modality. We could not address this question for the raw score versus standard score and the immediate versus maintenance assessment comparisons because virtually no studies used standard scores as dependent variables or tested for maintenance of effects.

Permutation tests indicated that the probability of strong evidence of a treatment effect did not vary by type of evidence of language development ($p = .27$), the most frequent two aspects of language measured (i.e., vocabulary and grammar; $p = .08$), or whether the outcome was specific to and the same aspect of language as the language target ($p = .08$). However, language intervention was more likely to affect the production measures (62%; 59/95) than the comprehension measures (25%; 3/12; $p = .03$).

Permutation tests indicated that adjusted effect size did not vary by type of evidence of language development ($p = .18$), the most frequent aspects of language (i.e., vocabulary vs. grammar) ($p = .47$), or degree to which the outcome matched the language target ($p = .89$). However, the average effect size on production measures (mean = 1.14; $SD = .60$) was larger than that on comprehension measures (mean = .59; $SD = .61$; $p = .01$).

Focused Analysis on Strong Evidence of Language Development

Similar findings were found when we focus our analysis only on the two classes of dependent variables that constitute relatively strong evidence of language development (i.e., conceptual reorganization and generalization to conversation). There was strong evidence of a treatment effect for 61% (31) of the effects tested. The average adjusted effect size for only these dependent variables was 1.14 ($SD = .56$).

DISCUSSION

This best-evidence review revealed that the majority of effects tested showed strong evidence of a treatment effect and that the average adjusted effect size was over 1.0. This average effect size exceeds what Cohen (1988) called a large effect size for behavioral research. These conclusions hold even when looking only at the effects that provide relatively strong evidence of language development. The average size of the treatment effect was largest for production measures. The probability of a treatment effect was highest for child oriented treatments, production measures, and randomized between-group experiments.

It is tempting to use the association between treatment effects and research design, treatment orientation or modality of outcome to draw conclusions about the types of research design, treatments, and dependent variables that yield the best results. However, it should be noted that these variables may vary with other potentially important variables that we did not examine. Like most literature reviews, the research design for this review is a correlational one. Correlational designs do not allow confident, causal explanations for the observed associations.

For example, the finding that randomized between-group designs are associated with better results should not be interpreted as suggesting that randomized group designs are to be favored when testing the efficacy of treatments. The association between research design and probability of treatment effects may have been due to unmeasured third variables. However, two explanations for the association between probability of a treatment effect and research design can be rejected. First, it is clear that the use of statistics is not sufficient to explain the association between treatment effects and the use of randomized between-group experiments. Otherwise, pre-post experiments with nonsense words would have been equally likely to be associated with probability of treatment effects. Second, it is clear that randomized between-group experiments did not have more production measures or more child oriented treatments than other designs in the review (chi square = 1.5 and 3.2; p = .47 and .20, respectively).

Additionally, the precise interpretation of results varies as a function of the research design. The results of randomized group experiments tell us about the performance of groups as a function of treatment. The results of single-subject experiments tell us about the performance of an individual as a function of treatment. Finally, pre-post designs with nonsense or unfamiliar words tell us about language acquisition without the benefit of transactions outside of the treatment session. Therefore, the selection of research design should be, in part, determined by the investigator's purpose, not by the hope that randomized group experiments will be more likely to yield expected findings.

It is useful to consider the association between treatment effect and modality of outcome and treatment orientation as the basis for hypothesis generation. To test these hypotheses, we need to manipulate modality of outcome and treatment orientation in the context of an internally valid study that controls all other variables.

Some internally valid studies have compared child oriented and adult oriented treatments. Camarata, Nelson, and Camarata (1994) compared conversational recasting (a child oriented approach) with imitation training in a didactic format (an adult oriented approach) in preschoolers with PLD. The results showed that recasts facilitated generalization of grammatical targets faster than imitation training. However, others who have compared a child oriented approach (i.e., Milieu teaching) and an adult oriented approach (i.e., a drill and practice approach) in children with intellectual disabilities have found that the relative efficacy of the treatments varied as a function of the pre-treatment developmental level of the children (Yoder, Kaiser, and Alpert 1991). The possibility that the relative efficacy of child versus adult oriented treatments varies by child developmental level needs to be tested in children with PLD.

Additionally, it should be noted that in both of the above studies many aspects of the treatments varied, not just whether the treatments were child or adult oriented. A more informative test of the hypothesis that a child oriented or hybrid treatment is more effective or more efficient than an adult oriented treatment needs to equate the treatments on all other aspects of the treatments. Among variables are (a) number of trials, (b) presence and method of eliciting child production of platform utterances or language targets, and (c) presence and type of linguistic consequences to child talk.

A study that did control for these variables while testing the relative efficacy of teaching to the child's focus of attention versus teaching to the adult's focus of attention was conducted with children with intellectual disabilities (Yoder et al. 1993). The study found that teaching to the child's attentional focus was more efficient than the adult asking the child to follow the adult's agenda when teaching object labels. However, we do not know if this pattern of results generalizes to children with PLD or to facilitating other aspects of language in addition to object labels.

To make the comparison of efficacy for comprehension versus production measures, we need to control for the aspect and level of specificity of language outcome, the treatment, and the participants. A look at three such studies with children with PLD reveals conflicting results. Such comparisons have found treatment effects on (a) production, but not comprehension (Connell 1986a; Gibbard 1994, experiment 2 for parent implemented treatment), (b) both production and comprehension to an extent (Gibbard 1994, experiment 1), (c) neither production nor comprehension using global measures of language (Gibbard 1994; experiment 2 for the individual treatment model). A sound meta-analysis of studies would require more studies with these controls.

If more sound studies that allow direct comparisons of treatment effects on production and comprehension measures confirm the finding in this review, one possible explanation is that comprehension measures are less direct reflections of language ability than production measures and are, therefore, more subject to measurement error (Tomasello and Mervis 1994). Measurement error usually increases the probability of missing treatment effects that would be detected with better measures (type II errors). Greater error in comprehension measures could explain the association between the probability of treatment effects and modality of outcome. However, at present, the literature does not allow definitive conclusions about the relative efficacy of language intervention for production versus comprehension measures.

It is clear that we need more studies on the efficacy of treatment for comprehension measures. Only 6 of the 23 studies included any comprehension measures (Rice, Buhr, and Nemeth 1990; Schwartz 1988; Connell 1986a; Gibbard 1994, studies 1 and 2; Connell and Stone 1992), and only two of these showed strong evidence of a treatment effect on the comprehension measure (Gibbard 1994, study 1; Rice, Buhr, and Nemeth 1990). Better measures of comprehension may improve our ability to detect treatment effects on comprehension.

The lack of information on the maintenance of treatment effects over months or years after the end of the treatment phase is a serious omission in the literature. Without such maintenance of effects, it could be argued that treatment is worthless. It should be noted that we are not saying that treatment has no long-term effect on language development. We are saying that maintenance of treatment effects has not been tested in the context of an internally valid treatment study of young children with primary language disorders. In this era of accountability, it is imperative that maintenance of results be tested in the near future.

In summary, this review found replicated evidence that language interventions tend to result in at least short-term, large gains in language development in preschoolers and toddlers with PLD. Hypotheses about the most effective treatments and most easily affected modality of language were suggested because greater gains were found when using child oriented treatments and when using production measures. Future work is needed to (a) test these hypotheses, (b) develop better comprehension measures, and (c) measure the long-term effects of language intervention.

REFERENCES

American Psychiatric Association. 2000. *Diagnostic and Statistical Manual of Mental Disorders, Fourth Edition, Text Revision.* Washington, DC: American Psychiatric Association.

Camarata, S. M. 1993. The application of naturalistic conversation training to speech production in children with speech disabilities. *Journal of Applied Behavior Analysis* 26:173–82.

Camarata, S. M., Nelson, K. E., and Camarata, M. N. 1994. Comparison of conversational recasting and imitative procedures for training grammatical structures in children with specific language impairment. *Journal of Speech and Hearing Research* 37:1414–23.

Cohen, J. 1988. *Statistical Power Analysis,* (2nd edition). Hillsdale, NJ: Erlbaum.

Connell, P. J. 1986a. Acquisition of semantic role by language-disordered children: Differences between production and comprehension. *Journal of Speech and Hearing Research* 29:366–74.

Connell, P. J. 1986b. Teaching subjecthood to language-disordered children. *Journal of Speech and Hearing Research* 29:481–92.

Connell, P. J. 1987. An effect of modeling and imitation teaching procedures on children with and without specific language impairment. *Journal of Speech and Hearing Research* 30:105–13.

Connell, P. J., and Stone, C. A. 1992. Morpheme learning of children with specific language impairment under controlled instructional conditions. *Journal of Speech and Hearing Research* 35:844–52.

Conti-Ramsden, G., and Botting, N. 2000. Educational placements for children with specific language impairments. In *Speech and Language Impairments in Children: Causes, Characteristics, Intervention and Outcome* (pp. 211–225), eds. D. V. M. Bishop and L. B. Leonard. Philadelphia, PA: Psychology Press.

Cooper, J., Moodley, M., and Reynell, J. 1979. The developmental language programme. Results from a five year study. *British Journal of Disorders of Communication* 14:57–69.

Courtright, J. A., and Courtright, I. C. 1976. Imitative modeling as a theoretical base for instructing language-disordered children. *Journal of Speech and Hearing Research* 19:655–63.

Culatta, B., and Horn, D. 1982. A program for achieving generalization of grammatical rules to spontaneous discourse. *Journal of Speech and Hearing Disorders* 47:174–80.

Dollagen, C., and Kaston, N. 1986. A comprehension monitoring program for language-impaired children. *Journal of Speech and Hearing Disorders* 51:264–71.

Dunn, L. M., and Dunn, L. M. 1997. *Peabody Picture Vocabulary Test.* Circle Pines, MN: American Guidance Service.

Edgington, E. S. 1984. Statistics and single case analysis. In *Progress in Behavior Modification: Vol. 16* (pp 83–120), eds. M. Hersen, R. M. Eisler, and P. M. Miller. New York: Raven Press.

Evesham, M. 1977. Teaching language skills to children with language disorders. *British Journal of Disorders of Communication* 12:23–29.

Ferron, J., and Onghena, P. 1996. Analyzing single case data: The power of randomization tests. *Journal of Experimental Education* 63:167–78.

Fey, M. In press. Ten principles of grammar facilitation for children with specific language impairments. In *Interdisciplinary Approaches to Specific Language Impairment*, ed. R. G. Schwartz. Hillsdale, NJ: Erlbaum.

Fey, M. E., Cleave, P. L., Long, S. H., and Hughes, D. L. 1993. Two approaches to the facilitation of grammar in children with language impairment: An experimental evaluation. *Journal of Speech and Hearing Research* 36:141–57.

Fey, M., and Proctor-Williams, K. 2000. Recasting, elicited imitation and modeling in grammar intervention for children with specific language impairments. In *Speech and Language Impairments in Children: Causes, Characteristics, Intervention and Outcome* (pp. 177–194), eds. D. V. M. Bishop and L. B. Leonard. Philadelphia, PA: Psychology Press.

Gardner, M. P. 1990. *Expressive One-Word Picture Vocabulary Test.* Austin, TX: PRO-ED.

Gibbard, D. 1994. Parental based intervention with preschool language-delayed children. *European Journal of Disorders of Communication* 29:131–50.

Gierut, J. A. 1990. Differential learning of phonological oppositions. *Journal of Speech and Hearing Research* 33:540–49.

Girolametto, L., Pearce, P. S., and Weitzman, E. 1996a. The effects of focused stimulation for promoting vocabulary in young children with delays: A pilot study. *Journal of Children's Communication Development* 17:39–49.

Girolametto, L., Pearce, P. S., and Weitzman, E. 1996b. Interactive focused stimulation for toddlers with expressive vocabulary delays. *Journal of Speech and Hearing Research* 39:1274–83.

Girolametto, L., Pearce, P. S., and Weitzman, E. 1997. Effects of lexical intervention on the phonology of late talkers. *Journal of Speech and Hearing Research* 40:338–48.

Glogowska, M., Roulstone, S., Enderby, P., and Peters, T. 2000. Randomised controlled trial of community based speech and language therapy in preschool children. *British Medical Journal* 321:1–5.

Good, P. I. 2000. *Permutation Tests: A Practical Guide to Resampling Methods for Testing Hypotheses.* New York: Springer.

Gottsleben, R. H., Tyack, D., and Buschini, G. 1974. Three case studies in language training: Applied linguistics. *Journal of Speech and Hearing Disorders* 39:213–24.

Hart, B., and Risley, T. 1995. *Meaningful Differences in the Everyday Experiences of Young American Children.* Baltimore, MD: Paul H. Brookes.

Hayes, A. 1996. Permutation test is not distribution-free: Testing the null hypothesis: $p = 0$. *Psychological Methods* 1:184–98.

Hedge, M. N., and Gierut, J. 1979. The operant training and generalization of pronouns and a verb form in a language-delayed child. *Journal of Communication Disorders* 12:23–34.

Hedge, M. N., Noll, M. J., and Pecora, R. 1979. A study of some factors affecting generalization of language training. *Journal of Speech and Hearing Disorders* 44:293–300.

Hegdes, L. V. 1981. Distribution theory for Glass's estimator of effect size and related estimators. *Journal of Educational Statistics* 6:107–28.

Hester, P., and Hendrickson, J. 1977. Training functional expressive language: The acquisition and generalization of five element syntactic responses. *Journal of Applied Behavior Analysis* 10: 316.

Johnston, J., Blatchley, M., and Olness, G. S. 1990. Miniature language system acquisition by children with different learning proficiencies. *Journal of Speech and Hearing Research* 33:335–42.

Kaiser, A. P., Hemmeter, M. L., Ostrosky, M. M., Alpert, C. L., and Hancock, T. B. 1995. The effects of group training and individual feedback on parent use of milieu teaching. *Journal of Childhood Communication Disorders* 16:39–48.

Kamhi, A. 1988. A reconceptualization of generalization and generalization problems. *Language, Speech, & Hearing Services in Schools* 19:314–29.

Law, J., Boyle, J., Harris, F., Harkness, A., and Nye, C. 1998. Screening for speech and language delay: A systematic review of the literature. *Health Technology Assessment* 9(2).

Leonard, L. B. 1982. Early lexical acquisition in children with specific language impairment. *Journal of Speech and Hearing Research* 25:554–64.

Leonard, L. B. 1998. The nature and efficacy of treatment. In *Children with Specific Language Impairment* (pp. 193–210) ed. L. B. Leonard. Cambridge, MA: MIT Press.

Leonard, L. B., Schwartz, R. G., Allen, G. D., Swanson, L. A., and Loeb, D. F. 1989. Unusual phonological behavior and the avoidance of homonymy in children. *Journal of Speech and Hearing Research* 32:583–90.

Leonard, L. B., Schwartz, R. G., Chapman, K., Rowan, L. E., Prelock, P. A., Terrell, B., Weiss, A. L., and Messick, C. 1982. Early lexical acquisition in children with specific language impairment. *Journal of Speech and Hearing Research* 25:554–64.

Levin, J. R., Marascuilo, L. A., and Hubert, L. J. 1978. N= nonparametric randomization tests. In *Single Subject Research: Strategies for Evaluating Change* (pp. 167–196), ed. T. R. Kratochwill. New York: Academic Press.

Lieberman, D. A. 1993. *Learning, Behavior, and Cognition.* Pacific Grove, CA: Brooks/Cole.

Lipsey, M., and Wilson, D. 2001. *Practical Meta-analysis.* Thousand Oaks, CA: Sage Publications.

Matheny, N., and Panagos, J. M. 1978. Comparing the effects of articulation and syntax programs on syntax and articulation improvement. *Language, Speech and Hearing Services in Schools* 9:50–56.

McCormick, L., and Schiefelbusch, R. 1990. *Early Language Intervention: An Introduction* (2nd edition). Columbus, OH: Merrill Publishing Company.

McGregor, K. K. 1994. Use of phonological information in a word-finding treatment for children. *Journal of Speech and Hearing Research* 37:1381–93.

McGregor, K. K., and Leonard, L. B. 1989. Facilitating word-finding skills of language impaired children. *Journal of Speech and Hearing Disorders* 54:141–47.

Miller, J. 1999. Profiles of language development in children with Down syndrome. In *Improving the Communication of People with Down Syndrome* (pp. 11 39), eds. J. Miller, M. Leddy, and L. Leavitt. Baltimore: Paul H. Brookes.

Nelson, K. E., 1989. Strategies for first language teaching. In *The Teachability of Language* (pp. 263 310), eds. M. Rice and R. Schiefelbusch. Baltimore: Paul H. Brookes.

Nelson, K. E., Camarata, S. M., Welsh, J., Butkovky, L., and Camarata, M. 1996. Effects of imitative and conversational recasting treatment on the acquisition of grammar in children with specific language impairment and younger language-normal children. *Journal of Speech and Hearing Research* 39:850–59.

Olswang, L. B., and Bain, B. A. 1985. Monitoring phoneme acquisition for making treatment withdrawal decisions. *Applied Psycholinguistics* 6:17–37.

Olswang, L. B., Bain, B. A., Dunn, C., and Cooper, J. 1983. The effects of stimulus variation on lexical learning. *Journal of Speech and Hearing Disorders* 48:192–201.

Olswang, L. B., Bain, B. A., Rosendahl, P. D., Oblak, S. B., and Smith, A. E. 1986. Language learning: Moving performance from a context dependent to independent state. *Child Language Teaching and Therapy* 2:180–210.

Olswang, L. B., and Coggins, T. E. 1984. The effects of adult behaviors on increasing language delayed children's production of early relational meanings. *British Journal of Disorders of Communication* 19:15–34.

Pearce, P., Girolametto, L., and Weitzman, E. 1996. The effects of focused stimulation intervention mothers of late-talking toddlers. *Infant Toddler Intervention* 6:213–27.

Pinker, S. 1994. *The Language Instinct: How the Mind Creates Language.* New York: Morrow.

Reynell, J., and Gruber, C. 1990. *Reynell Developmental Language Scales.* Los Angeles, CA: Western Psychological Services.

Rice, M. L., Buhr, J. C., and Nemeth, M. 1990. Fast mapping word learning abilities of language delayed preschoolers. *Journal of Speech and Hearing Research* 55:33–42.

Rice, M. L., Sell, M. A., and Hadley, P. A. 1990. The social interactive coding system (SICS): An on-line, clinically relevant descriptive tool. *Language, Speech, and Hearing Services in Schools* 21:2–14.

Robertson, S. B., and Weismer, S. E. 1997. The influence of peer models on the play scripts of children with specific language impairment. *Journal of Speech and Hearing Research* 40:49–61.

Robertson, S. B., and Weismer, S. E. 1999. Effects of treatment on linguistic and social skills in toddlers with delayed language development. *Journal of Speech and Hearing Research* 42:1234–48.

Roseberry, C. A., and Connell, P. J. 1991. The use of an invented language rule in the differentiation of normal and language-impaired Spanish-speaking children. *Journal of Speech and Hearing Research* 34:596–603.

Schwartz, R. G. 1988. Early action word acquisition in normal and language impaired children. *Applied Psycholinguistics* 9:110–22.

Schwartz, R. G., Chapman, K., Terrell, B. Y., Prelock, P., and Rowan, L. 1985. Facilitating word combination in language impaired children through discourse structure. *Journal of Speech and Hearing Disorders* 50:31–39.

Schwartz, R. G., Leonard, L. B., Messick, C., and Chapman, K. 1987. The acquisition of object names in children with specific language impairment: Action context and word extension. *Applied Psycholinguistics* 8:233–44.

Slavin, R. E. 1986. Best-evidence synthesis: An alternative to meta-analytic and traditional reviews. In *Evaluation Studies: Annual Review, Vol. 12* (pp. 667–673) eds. W. R. Shadish, Jr. and C. S. Reichardt. Thousand Oaks, CA: Sage Publications.

Sorensen, P., and Fey, M. E. 1992. Informativeness as a clinical principle: What's really new? *Journal of Speech and Hearing Research* 23:320–28.

Stark, R. E., and Tallal, P. 1981. Selection of children with specific language deficits. *Journal of Communication Disorders* 7:295–304.

Swisher, L., Restrepo, M. A., Plante, E., and Lowell, S. 1995. Effect of implicit and explicit "rule" presentation on bound morpheme generalization in specific language impairment. *Journal of Speech and Hearing Research* 38:168–73.

Swisher, L., and Snow, D. 1994. Learning and generalization components of morphological acquisition by children with specific language impairment: Is there a functional relation? *Journal of Speech and Hearing Research* 37:1406–13.

Tallal, P., Miller, S. L., Bedi, G., Byrna, G., Wang, X., Nagarajan, S. S., Schriener, C., Jenkins, W. M., and Merzenich, M. M. 1996. Language comprehension in language-learning impaired children improved with acoustically modified speech. *Science* 271:81–84.

Tomasello, M., and Mervis, C. 1994. The instrument is great, but measuring comprehension is still a problem. In *Variability in Early Communicative Development* (pp. 174–179), eds. L. Fenson, P. Dale, J. S. Reznick, E. Bates, D. Thal, and S. Pethnick. *Monographs of the Society for Research in Child Development* 224.

Warren, S. 1988. A behavioral approach to language generalization. *Language, Speech, & Hearing Services in Schools* 19:292–303.

Warren, S. F. and Kaiser, A. P. 1986. Generalization of treatment effects by young language-delayed children: A longitudinal analysis. *Journal of Speech and Hearing Disorders* 51:239–51.

Weismer, S. E. 2000. Intervention for children with developmental language delay. In *Speech and Language Impairments in Children: Causes, Characteristics, Intervention and Outcome* (pp. 157–176), eds. D. V. M. Bishop and L. B. Leonard. Philadelphia, PA: Psychology Press.

Weismer, S. E., and Murray-Branch, J. 1989. Modeling versus modeling plus evoked production training: A comparison of two language intervention methods. *Journal of Speech and Hearing Disorders* 54:269–81.

Weismer, S. E., Murray-Branch, J., and Miller, J. F. 1993. Comparison of two methods for promoting productive vocabulary in late talkers. *Journal of Speech and Hearing Research* 36: 1037–50.

Whitehurst, G. J., Fischel, J. E., Caulfield, M., DeBaryshe, B. D., and Valdez-Menchaca, M. C. 1989. Assessment and treatment of early expressive language delay. In *Challenges to Developmental Paradigms: Implications for Theory, Assessment and Treatment*, eds. Philip Zelazo and Ronald Barr. Hillsdale, NJ: Erlbaum.

Whitehurst, G. J., Novak, G., and Zorn, G. A. 1972. Delayed speech studied in the home. *Developmental Psychology* 7(2):169–77.

Wilcox, J. J., Kouri, T. A., and Caswell, S. B. 1991. Early language intervention: A comparison of classroom and individual treatment. *American Journal of Speech Language Pathology* 49–62.

Wilcox, M. J., and Leonard, L. B. 1978. Experimental acquisition of wh-questions in language disordered children. *Journal of Speech and Hearing Research* 21:220–39.

Wing, C. S. 1990. A preliminary investigation of generalization to untrained words following two treatments of children's word finding problems. *Language, Speech and Hearing Services in Schools* 21:151–56.

Yoder, P. J., Kaiser, A. P., and Alpert, C. 1991. An exploratory study of the interaction between language teaching methods and child characteristics. *Journal of Speech and Hearing Research* 34:155–67.

Yoder, P. J., Kaiser, A. P., Alpert, C., and Fischer, R. 1993. The effect of following the child's lead on the efficiency of teaching nouns with preschoolers with mental retardation. *Journal of Speech and Hearing Research* 36:158–67.

Zwitman, D. H., and Sonderman, J. C. 1979. A syntax program designed to present base linguistic structures to language disordered children. *Journal of Communication Disorders* 12:323–35.

Appendix A.   Rejected Studies by Rationale for Rejection

Citation	Population characteristics				Internal validity	Comments
	Nonverbal IQ	No Expressive Delay	Hearing screening passed?	CA		
Olswang & Bain (1985)		XX				Expressive language within normal limits
Weismer & Murray Branch (1989)					XX	Alternating treatment design with same targets used for both intervention phases
Olswang, Bain, Dunn & Cooper (1983)					XX	Did not test development; No generalization across person/material
Camarata (1993)		XX				No language testing data reported; only articulation test results
Girolametto, Pearce & Weitzman, (1996a)	XX					Subjects did not meet nonverbal IQ criteria
Wilcox, Kouri, & Caswell, (1991)	XX					IQ data given for group, not individuals; Mean DQ for Individual Group =.72; Mean DQ for Classroom Group = .81
Connell (1987)		XX				Unclear if S's meet expressive delay of 1.25 SD or 70% of CA
McGregor (1994)		XX		XX		Expressive language criterion unclear; No morphology/ syntax measures
Johnston, Blatchley, & Olness (1990)				XX		Age range 7–8 to 9–10
McGregor & Leonard (1989)				XX		Age range 9–1 to 10–5
Dollaghan & Kaston (1986)				XX		Age range 5–10 to 8–2
Gottsleben, Tyack & Buschini (1974)				XX		Age range 7–9 yrs
Wing (1990)					XX	Age range 71–85 months

Citation	Population characteristics				Internal validity	Comments
	Nonverbal IQ	No Expressive Delay	Hearing screening passed?	CA		
Hegde, Noll & Pecora (1979)	XX					CA=3–9; PPVT MA=2–2; DQ=26/45=.58
Courtright & Courtright (1976)		XX		XX		No expressive language scores given; Age range 5–10 years
Matheny & Panagos (1978)	XX			XX		Age range 65–82 months; No receptive language or IQ measure
Kaiser, Hemmeter, Ostrosky, Alpert & Hancock (1995)					XX	
Gierut (1990)		XX				Subjects have phonological impairments only; do not meet criteria for expressive delay
Nelson, Camarata, Welsh, Butkovsky & Camarata (1996)				XX		3/7 PLD subjects CA > 73 months
Roseberry & Connell (1991)						Subjects are bilingual
Sorensen & Fey (1992)					XX	No data by session; data summarized by frequency of target production; not possible to evaluate change in slope or to compare informative vs. redundant interaction style
Pearce, Girolametto & Weitzman (1996)	XX					No nonverbal IQ score; used receptive language age to compute IQ; 50% of sample had DQ<.70
Glogowska et al (2000)	Unclear	Unclear	7/21 had diag-nosed loss			Types of language delay in experimental group unclear

Citation	Population characteristics				Internal validity	Comments
	Nonverbal IQ	No Expressive Delay	Hearing screening passed?	CA		
Rice, Sell & Hadley (1990)		XX				4/7 language impaired subjects do not meet criterion for expressive delay: these S's have numerous articulation errors and expressive skills < 1.25 SD below mean for age
Tallal et. al. (1996)				XX	XX	No random assignment; used controls matched for nonverbal IQ & receptive language level; Mean CA = 7.4 yrs
Zwitman & Sonderman (1979)		XX				No standardized expressive language information provided
Eversham (1977)				XX		No CA's given
Leonard, Schwartz, Allen, Swanson & Loeb (1989)					XX	No statistical results given
Hester & Hendrickson (1977)					XX	Insufficient data
Connell (1986b)					XX	Pre-experimental design
Warren & Kaiser (1986)					XX	
Culatta & Horn (1982)		XX	Not specified	XX		Too old; no language delay
Cooper, Moodley & Reynell (1979)	XX					Cognitive status unclear
Schwartz, Chapman, Terrell, Prelock, & Rowan, 1985					XX	Pre/post design with no control group and early words
Whitehurst, Novak, & Zorn (1972)					XX	AB with reversal
Leonard, 1982		XX				

Chapter • 10

Language and Academic Outcomes of Children with Preschool Language Disorders

Carla J. Johnson and Joseph H. Beitchman

What becomes of children with language disorders as they grow up? Do they outgrow their difficulties or do problems persist? If the latter, what domains of functioning are affected and to what extent? Answers to these questions are crucial to the development of appropriate intervention strategies and public policies to support such children, their families, and their communities.

OVERVIEW OF THE OTTAWA LANGUAGE STUDY (OLS)

The Ottawa Language Study (OLS) addressed these key questions on the long-term outcomes of children with preschool language disorders. The OLS began in 1982 with a large-scale speech/language screening of a 1-in-3 stratified sample of children ($n = 1655$) from English-language schools in the Ottawa-Carleton region of Ontario, Canada (Beitchman, Nair, Clegg, and Patel 1986). Children who failed the screening received comprehensive speech/language assessments, as did a random sample of children who passed the screening.

A group of 142 children with identified speech/language disorders (the S/L group) then participated in a further longitudinal portion of the study. This S/L group was matched on age, sex, and school to a control group of 142 children without disorders. The full longitudinal sample ($n = 284$) then received further assessments, which included measures of demographic information, medical history, psychosocial functioning, cognitive performance, and parental mental health. Results of this Time 1 portion of the OLS are described in detail elsewhere (Beitchman, Hood, Rochon, and Peterson 1989; Beitchman, Hood, Rochon et al. 1989; Beitchman, Nair, Clegg, Ferguson, and Patel 1986; Beitchman, Nair, Clegg, and Patel 1986).

Comprehensive follow-up assessments (Times 2 and 3) also took place when participants in the longitudinal sample were 12 and 19 years old, respectively. Results for Time 2 are reported elsewhere (Beitchman et al. 1994; Beitchman, Brownlie et al. 1996; Beitchman, Wilson, Brownlie, Walters, Inglis et al. 1996; Beitchman, Wilson, Brownlie, Walters, and Lancee 1996).

This chapter will focus on the results of the Time 3 follow-up that took place when participants were 19 years of age. The primary emphasis will be on the language and academic outcomes of the children with language disorders at age five. Outcomes for this group will be compared to those for two other groups: children with early speech-only disorders and children without early speech or language disorders.

THE LONGITUDINAL SAMPLE

To understand the Time 3 outcomes, it is necessary to have a clear picture of the Time 1 longitudinal sample, and, in particular, of the 142 children with speech/language disorders (S/L group). A subset of these children ($n = 39$) had one or more speech-only disorders (e.g., articulation, fluency, voice) at age five. Most children in this speech-only subgroup had articulation disorders, as indicated by Time 1 performance more than two standard deviations below the mean on the Word Articulation subtest of the Test of Language Development (Newcomer and Hammill 1977). Fluency and voice disorders were identified via clinical judgments made by the speech-language pathologists who conducted the speech-language evaluations.

A larger subset of the S/L group ($n = 103$) presented with language disorders at age five, either with ($n = 41$) or without ($n = 62$) accompanying speech disorders. These children performed more than one standard deviation below the mean on one or more of several standardized language tests, primarily the Test of Language Development (Newcomer and Hammill 1977) and the Peabody Picture Vocabulary Test Revised (Dunn and Dunn 1981). Language disorders were identified solely on the basis of performance on standardized language tests (Lahey 1990). No exclusionary criteria or cognitive referencing standards were applied. Thus, this OLS subgroup included children whose language disorders occurred in either the absence or the presence of concomitant sensory, structural, neurological, or cognitive conditions.

IMPORTANCE OF THE OLS

The OLS is important because it incorporates a unique combination of desirable methodological features not found in other follow-up studies of adults with histories of speech/language disorders (Felsenfeld, Broen, and McGue 1992, 1994; Hall and Tomblin 1978; King, Jones, and Lasky 1982; Lewis and Freebairn 1992; Tomblin, Freese, and Records 1992). A key feature of the OLS is its prospective nature, with both S/L and control groups identified at the start of the study and followed forward in time. Most other follow-up studies of young adults used a retrospective design, in which controls were not identified at the same time as cases, thereby limiting possible conclusions. The OLS is also the longest prospective study available in the literature, spanning a period of 14 years, from ages 5 to 19. Moreover, the children in the OLS comprised a community sample, thereby avoiding potential biases that may affect clinic-referred samples. Participants also presented with a variety of speech/language disorders, representative in both severity and type of those found in the population. Finally, the OLS incorporated direct testing of multiple domains of functioning at each time period, including speech/language, cognitive, academic, psychosocial/behavioral, demographic, and parental mental health. Taken together, these desirable design features lend confidence to the findings and conclusions of the OLS.

TIME 3 PARTICIPANTS

It is notoriously difficult, albeit essential, to keep in touch with participants over the course of longitudinal studies because they move, change names, or both. At Time 3, the OLS investigators collected at least some data from more than 90% of the original 284 study participants. Only 7 refused to participate; 17 could not be located; and 2 had died since the start of the study, 14 years earlier.

Special efforts helped to ensure this high participation rate. The research team relied on tips from relatives and friends as well as Internet and telephone directory searches to locate participants. Although most testing took place in the Ottawa-Carleton area where the study originated, additional testing teams in Toronto and Vancouver evaluated participants who had moved to those cities.

Telephone testing permitted the participation of those who lived in other countries or remote locations in Canada. If necessary, testing was completed in participants' homes or in prisons or detention centers. In one case, a participant escaped from prison, forcing the testing team to postpone its assessment until he was recaptured!

Information in this chapter is based on 242 of the original participants (85%) for whom complete speech/language data were collected at Time 3. These participants included 114 from the original S/L group and 128 from the original control group. Their mean age at Time 3 testing was 18 years, 11 months. The sample was 65% male and 45% high SES (Blishen, Carroll, and Moore 1987). Approximately 75% were enrolled in school (high school, community college, or university) and about 59% had full- or part-time jobs (Johnson, Beitchman et al. 1999).

Those who participated at Time 3 appeared to be representative of their original S/L and control groups. Specifically, participants and non-participants did not differ significantly on most age 5 characteristics. Thus, results from the Time 3 participants can be generalized with confidence to the original population from which they were selected.

TIME 3 ASSESSMENTS

Each Time 3 participant completed an individual battery of measures that took approximately six hours to administer. A speech-language pathologist conducted 1.5 hours of speech/language assessments; a psychometrist administered 2 hours of cognitive and academic achievement measures; and a trained interviewer collected 2.5 hours of demographic, psychosocial, and behavioral information. The research team also gathered parent and teacher reports of participants' psychosocial/behavioral characteristics as well as parental reports of their own mental health. Multiple measures typically represented each domain of functioning. Measures were chosen to be age-appropriate and conceptually similar to those used at Times 1 and 2. The figure captions in this chapter include the names of the specific Time 3 measures upon which the depicted results are based.

Space limitations preclude a full presentation of OLS findings here. Thus, we will address three main questions of interest. First, we will provide an overview of Time 3 functional outcomes in various domains for the two original S/L and control groups. We will then narrow our focus to discussion of language and academic outcomes particularly for the subset of children with histories of language disorder. We will compare outcomes for these children to those for children from two other groups: those with histories of speech-only disorders and those who did not have speech or language disorders at age 5. Finally, we will present information on speech-language interventions that occurred during the course of the 14-year OLS. Unfortunately, given the design of the OLS, it is not possible to determine the efficacy of those interventions.

COMPARISON OF FUNCTIONAL OUTCOMES FOR ORIGINAL S/L AND CONTROL GROUPS

We begin with an overview of functional outcomes at Time 3. Figure 1 shows the percentages of young adults from the original S/L and control groups who exhibited various adverse outcomes at Time 3. The outcomes shown include rates of: (a) communication disorders (speech and/or language), (b) reading disorders, (c) psychiatric diagnoses, (d) school drop out, and (e) arrests. For each of these adverse outcomes, the original S/L group showed significantly higher rates than the original control group. Further details on these adverse outcomes are available in other publications concerning the Time 3 OLS results (Beitchman, Adlaf et al. 2001; Beitchman et al. 1999; Beitchman, Wilson et al. 2001; Johnson, Beitchman et al. 1999; Young et al. 2002). For our purposes here, suffice it to say that it is clear that children with histories of early speech/language disorders are at heightened risk for adverse outcomes in a variety of domains compared to their peers without disorders.

LANGUAGE AND ACADEMIC OUTCOMES OF CHILDREN WITH LANGUAGE DISORDERS

Time 3 Rates of Communication Disorders

We now narrow our focus to the language and academic outcomes of young adults with early language disorders. Recall that at Time 1 roughly 75% of children in the original S/L group had language disorders (with or without accompanying speech disorders) and the remaining 25% had speech-only disorders. Figure 2 shows the rates of communication disorders at Time 3 for these two Time 1 subgroups and the original control group. Overall, individuals showed a strong tendency to continue in the same category. More than 70% of the individuals with language disorders at Time 1 also had language disorders at Time 3, as determined by performance more than one standard deviation below the mean on the published norms of the Peabody Picture Vocabulary Test Revised (Dunn and Dunn 1981) or on the

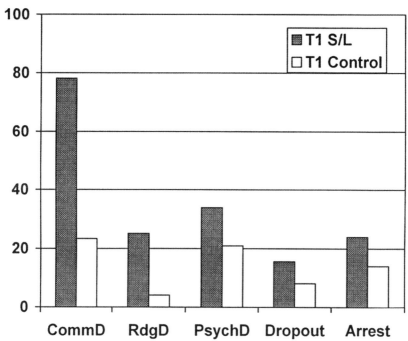

Figure 1 Time 3 Functional Outcome Rates (% of Participants) for the Time 1 (T1) Speech/Language (S/L) and Control Groups. CommD = communication disorders [language disorders or speech-only disorders; criterion for language disorder = test performance < 1 standard deviation below the mean on the Peabody Picture Vocabulary Test Revised (Dunn and Dunn 1981) or the local norms (Johnson, Taback et al. 1999) for the Spoken Language Quotient of the Test of Adolescent/Adult Language 3 (Hammill et al. 1994); criterion for speech-only disorder = judgment by speech-language pathologist]; RdgD = reading disorders [criterion = tested performance < 1 standard deviation below the mean on Broad Reading composite of Woodcock-Johnson Psychoeducational Battery Revised (Woodcock and Johnson 1989)]; PsychD = one or more psychiatric diagnoses [criterion = as identified by the University of Michigan version of the Composite International Diagnostic Interview (Kessler et al. 1994) plus a score < 70 on the Global Assessment of Functioning (American Psychiatric Association 1994)]; Dropout = school dropout [criterion = as reported by participants]; Arrest = arrested at least once [criterion = as reported by participants].

local norms (Johnson, Taback et al. 1999) for the Spoken Language Quotient of the Test of Adolescent/Adult Language 3 (Hammill et al. 1994). Similarly, more than 40% of those with speech-only disorders at Time 1 also had speech-only disorders at Time 3, as judged by the speech-language pathologist. As shown in each set of bars in Figure 2, these rates for persisting disorders far exceeded the Time 3 disorder

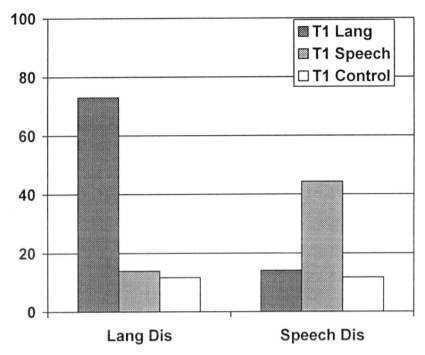

Figure 2. Time 3 Rates (% of Participants) of Language Disorders (Lang Dis) and Speech-only Disorders (Speech Dis) for the Three Time 1 (T1) Subgroups: Language Disorders (Lang), Speech-only Disorders (Speech) and Control.

rates for the respective Time 1 comparison groups, which did not differ significantly from each other.

We should also briefly describe the speech-only disorders identified at Time 3. They were usually articulation problems of a very mild nature that did not greatly reduce speech intelligibility. To illustrate, only one Time 3 participant received a rating of speech intelligibility that was less than 95% in conversation, as judged by the speech-language pathologist.

Standardized Tests of Language, Cognition, and Academic Achievement

Figure 3 compares the Time 3 performances of the three groups of interest on standardized measures of language, cognition, and academic achievement (reading, spelling, math). The patterns of results are strikingly consistent across all six measures. Young adults who had early language disorders performed markedly worse on all measures than those with early speech-only disorders or no disorders, whereas

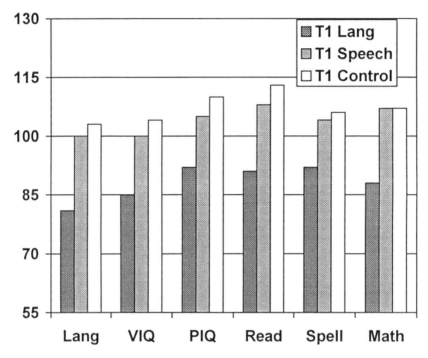

Figure 3.   Time 3 Performances (Standard Scores, M = 100, SD = 15) on Standardized Tests of Language (Lang), Verbal IQ (VIQ), Performance IQ (PIQ), and Academic Achievement in Reading (Read), Spelling (Spell), and Math for the Three Time 1 (T1) Subgroups: Language Disorders (Lang), Speech-only Disorders (Speech) and Control. Measures used were: Lang = local norms (Johnson, Taback et al. 1999) for the Spoken Language Quotient of the Test of Adolescent/Adult Language-3 (Hammill et al. 1994); VIQ and PIQ = short form version (Ward 1990) of the Wechsler Adult Intelligence Scale Revised (Wechsler 1981a); Read = Broad Reading composite of Woodcock-Johnson Psychoeducational Battery Revised (Woodcock and Johnson 1989); Spell = Spelling score of the Wide Range Achievement Test-3 (Wilkinson 1993); Math = Math Calculation score of Woodcock-Johnson Psycho-educational Battery Revised (Woodcock and Johnson 1989).

the latter two groups showed no significant differences from each other.

Criteria for Language Disorder

As mentioned earlier, the original criterion for language disorder used in the OLS was performance less than one standard deviation below the mean on one or more standardized language measures. The use of such a liberal criterion for disorder has drawn some criticism.

However, one advantage of using a liberal criterion initially in a longitudinal project is that one can then apply more stringent criteria in a post hoc fashion and evaluate the relative merits of the various cut-offs for specifying disorder (Aram, Ekelman, and Nation 1984). If a stringent criterion had been used initially, such an analysis would not be possible because participants who met the liberal criterion, but not the stringent one, would have been excluded from the study at the outset.

We took advantage of the opportunity afforded by the OLS to compare the effects of the original liberal criterion to those of a more stringent criterion, based on expert judgments from speech-language pathologists (Johnson, Beitchman et al. 1999). Application of the stringent criterion reduced the Time 1 prevalence of language disorders from 12.6% to 8.3%, but increased the Time 1 prevalence of speech-only disorders from 6.4% to 8.7%. The increase in speech-only disorders occurred because some participants who originally qualified as having both language and speech disorders no longer met the criterion for language disorders. An additional group of 21 individuals met the liberal but not the stringent criterion for language disorders. It was of particular interest to examine the long-term outcomes of these individuals whose tested language performance fell in the grey area between the two disorder criteria.

To do so, we completed analyses similar to those in figure 2 (Time 3 communication disorder rates) and figure 3 (Time 3 standardized test performance), but instead used four comparison groups based on application of the stringent criteria at Time 1 (language disorder, speech-only disorder, grey area, and control). Participants in the grey area did not fare particularly well at Time 3, while those in other disorder groups showed results remarkably similar to those shown earlier for the liberal criterion (Johnson, Beitchman et al. 1999). With respect to rates of communication disorders, about 40% of individuals in the grey area met the stringent criterion for language disorder at Time 3. As in the earlier analysis, roughly 70% of participants with initial language disorders and 40% of those with initial speech-only disorders demonstrated similar disorders at Time 3. On all standardized measures of language, cognition, and academic achievement, individuals in the grey area showed mean performances that were statistically indistinguishable from those of the language disorder group. The grey area and language disorder groups both performed more poorly than the speech-only and control groups, which did not differ from each other. The two criteria, therefore, yielded similar pictures of the long-term prognosis for children with early language disorders. In choosing a criterion, clinicians and researchers would need to weigh carefully the risks and benefits inherent in each choice.

Specific versus Secondary Language Disorders

At Time 1, the only criterion for identification of language disorder in the OLS was an inclusionary one, based entirely on standardized language test performance below a specified cut-off level. In the clinical and research literature, additional exclusionary criteria are often applied to distinguish those with specific language disorders (no exclusionary conditions) from those with language disorders thought to be secondary to the presence of one or more additional conditions (Stark and Tallal 1981). Some of the common exclusionary conditions include structural (e.g., cleft palate), sensory (e.g., hearing loss, blindness), neurological (e.g., epilepsy, cerebral palsy), or cognitive (e.g., autism, performance IQ < 80) impairments. Again, the inclusive nature of the OLS proved to be important, permitting us to make a retrospective examination of outcomes for individuals with specific versus secondary language disorders.

At Time 1, the ratio of individuals with specific to secondary language disorders in the OLS sample was approximately 5 to 1. By Time 3, this ratio had changed to roughly 2 to 1. A few participants acquired secondary impairments (e.g., due to late-onset hearing loss or traumatic brain injury) during the course of the 14-year study. However, declines in performance IQ to values below the cut-off of 80 accounted for the vast majority of new secondary impairments at Time 3. Similar declines in performance IQ have been reported in other follow-ups of children with histories of language disorder (Benasich, Curtiss, and Tallal 1993; Stothard et al. 1998; Tomblin et al. 1992). Interpretation of the OLS results, however, clearly demonstrated the importance of including a prospective control group in follow-up studies. Because similar declines in performance (and verbal) IQs also occurred in the OLS control group, it was clear that the phenomenon should not be interpreted as exclusive to those with language disorders. One possible explanation for the IQ declines is that they reflect differences in the two intelligence scales used at Time 1 and Time 3, the Wechsler Preschool and Primary Scale of Intelligence (Wechsler 1981b) and the short form version (Ward 1990) of the Wechsler Adult Intelligence Scale Revised (Wechsler 1981a).

We also compared Time 3 language disorder rates and standardized test performances for individuals with Time 1 specific versus secondary language disorders. The rates of persistent language disorder were similar for the two groups at slightly more than 70%. Standardized language test performances were significantly better, however, for those with specific as opposed to secondary language disorders. Thus, the overall long-term prognosis appeared to be somewhat better for those with specific as compared to secondary language disorders.

Self-Evaluations of Communication Skills

Another question of interest concerned the extent to which young adults with histories of language disorder were aware of their own communication difficulties. At Time 3, we asked participants to complete a 13-item self-evaluation checklist concerning their listening, speaking, reading, and writing skills (e.g., I read for pleasure whenever possible; I avoid getting involved in conversations and discussions). Most items were rated on a 4-point scale (1 = strongly agree, 2 = agree, 3 = disagree, 4 = strongly disagree).

The final item on this self-evaluation checklist required participants to give an overall evaluation of their communication skills. The exact wording for the item was "Overall, my communication abilities (listening, speaking, reading, writing) are. " Participants completed the item by rating their performance on a 7-point scale (1 = much poorer than average; 4 = average; 7 = much better than average). Figure 4 compares the rated and tested communication performances for the individuals with early language disorders to those from the speech-only and control groups. All groups showed a slight tendency to overrate their actual performance but this tendency was particularly pronounced for the individuals with early language disorders.

It is not clear exactly how to interpret this result. Does it mean that individuals with language disorders are unaware of their difficulties? Or is it possible that their typical peer group provides a different standard for comparison than that used by individuals in the other two groups? Children with language disorders may have immediate peer groups consisting of others with limited language skills. If so, the communication skills of those with language disorders may, indeed, be average relative to those of others in their peer reference groups.

Spontaneous Language Measures

We also wondered whether measures of spontaneous language performance at Time 3 would also distinguish the groups. The speech-language pathologist used a standard series of questions in a structured interview format to elicit a spontaneous language sample from each young adult participant. She also rated each interview for overall pragmatic quality (e.g., coherence, responsiveness) on a binary scale (0 = inadequate; 1 = adequate). The language samples were recorded for later transcription and analysis using the Systematic Analysis of Language Transcripts (SALT) software (Miller and Chapman 1997).

The interview samples averaged about 11 minutes in length. Table I shows comparisons of the samples from the three groups of

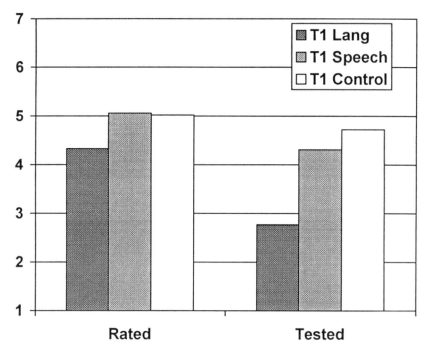

Figure 4. Time 3 Self-Ratings of Overall Communication Skills (1 = much poorer than average; 4 = average; 7 = much better than average) Compared to Tested Communication Performance [average of standard scores for the local norms (Johnson, Taback et al. 1999) for the Spoken Language Quotient of the Test of Adolescent/Adult Language-3 (Hammill et al. 1994) and the Broad Reading composite of Woodcock-Johnson Psychoeducational Battery Revised (Woodcock and Johnson 1989); average of test scores then converted to a 7 point scale in which the mean standard score of 100 = 4 and each standard score increment of 15 (1 standard deviation) = 1 scale point].

interest on a number of language characteristics. On the pragmatic quality measure, a familiar pattern emerges. Those with early language disorders show poorer quality ratings than those from the speech-only and control groups. The same pattern is apparent on the measure of vocabulary diversity, number of different words. The young adults with early language problems also produced shorter utterances than individuals from the control group, as indexed by mean length of t-unit (Hunt 1965). On a measure of speech rate, words per minute, the individuals with early speech disorders were significantly slower than were those from the control group.

Table I.   Selected Spontaneous Language Characteristics in Time 3 Interviews for the Three Time 1 (T1) Subgroups: Language Disorders (Lang), Speech-only Disorders (Speech) and Control.

Characteristic	T1 Lang	T1 Speech	T1 Control	Sig. Diffs.[a]
		Groups		
Quality Rating[b]	.64	.91	.88	L < S = C
MLTU[c]	7.67	8.32	8.69	L < C
Diff. Words[d]	329	344	393	L = S < C
Words/Minute	113	109	122	S < C

[a]Pattern of significant differences between T1 groups (L = Language Disorders; S = Speech-only Disorders; C = Control).

[b]Binary rating of pragmatic quality (e.g., cohesion, responsiveness) given by speech-language pathologist (1 = adequate; 0 = inadequate).

[c]Mean length of t-unit (Hunt 1965) in words.

[d]Number of different words.

Speech/Language Intervention

Approximately 50% of individuals in the original S/L group reportedly received speech-language intervention, usually during the first few years of the OLS when the children were in elementary grades. This relatively low overall rate of intervention occurred despite the fact that all parents of children in the Time 1 S/L group were given information on how and where to seek speech-language services. Because OLS participants were not randomly assigned to intervention, it was not possible to draw conclusions about the efficacy of the treatments they received.

It was possible, however, to examine the age 5 characteristics of those who did and did not receive speech-language interventions during the study. Children who received interventions showed poorer articulation abilities at age 5 than those who did not receive interventions, but the two groups did not differ significantly on measures of language ability, socioeconomic status, or performance IQ. In other words, the severity of speech difficulties was a major factor in determining which children were referred and accepted for speech-language intervention. In contrast, children with severe language disorders were not consistently identified as candidates for intervention. Tomblin et al. (1997) reported a similar result in a larger, more recent study, suggesting that the under-identification of children with severe language disorders is a persisting problem that has not been overcome since the early 1980s when the OLS began.

SUMMARY AND CONCLUSIONS

In young adulthood, children with early language disorders showed a wide range of adverse outcomes that are costly to individuals and society, in both human and financial terms. They exhibited high rates (70–75%) of persisting language disorder as well as poor outcomes in cognitive, academic, and psychosocial functioning. These adverse outcomes occurred at much higher rates for children with early language disorders than for those with early speech-only disorders. In fact, with the exception of modest rates of persistent mild speech difficulties, children with early speech disorders showed few, if any, adverse long-term outcomes. Yet, children with speech disorders were more likely than were those with language disorders to receive early intervention for their communication difficulties, a state of affairs that likely persists today.

The OLS findings highlight the need for much greater attention to the long-term, negative correlates of early language disorders. We need to intensify our efforts to identify such children early and to provide comprehensive interventions intended to maximize long-term outcomes across multiple domains of functioning.

REFERENCES

American Psychiatric Association 1994. *Diagnostic and Statistical Manual of Mental Disorders, 4th edition (DSM-IV)*. Washington, DC: American Psychiatric Association.

Aram, D. M., Ekelman, B., and Nation, J. 1984. Preschoolers with language disorders: Ten years later. *Journal of Speech and Hearing Research* 27:232–44.

Beitchman, J. H., Adlaf, E., Douglas, L., Atkinson, L., Young, A., Johnson, C. J., Escobar, M., and Wilson, B. 2001. Comorbidity of psychiatric and substance use disorders in late adolescence: A cluster analytic approach. *The American Journal of Drug and Alcohol Abuse* 27(3):421–40.

Beitchman, J. H., Brownlie, E. B., Inglis, A., Wild, J., Ferguson, B., Schachter, D., Lancee, W., Wilson, B., and Mathews, R. 1996. Seven-year follow-up of speech/language-impaired and control children: Psychiatric outcome. *Journal of Child Psychology and Psychiatry* 37:961–70.

Beitchman, J. H., Brownlie, E. B., Inglis, A., Wild, J., Mathews, R., Schachter, D., Kroll, R., Martin, S., Ferguson, B., and Lancee, W. 1994. Seven-year follow-up of speech/language-impaired and control children: Speech/language stability and outcome. *Journal of the American Academy of Child and Adolescent Psychiatry* 33:1323–30.

Beitchman, J. H., Douglas, L., Wilson, B., Johnson, C., Young, A., Atkinson, L., Escobar, M., and Taback, N. 1999. Adolescent substance use disorders: Findings from a 14-year follow-up of speech and language impaired and control children. *Journal of Child Clinical Psychology* 28:312–21.

Beitchman, J. H., Hood, J., Rochon, J., and Peterson, M. 1989. Empirical classification of speech/language impairment in children: II. Behavioral characteristics. *Journal of the American Academy of Child and Adolescent Psychiatry* 28:118–23.

Beitchman, J. H., Hood, J., Rochon, J., Peterson, M., Mantini, T., and Majumdar, S. 1989. Empirical classification of speech/language impairment in children: I. Identification of speech/language categories. *Journal of the American Academy of Child and Adolescent Psychiatry* 28:112–17.

Beitchman, J. H., Nair, R., Clegg, M., Ferguson, B., and Patel, P. G. 1986. Prevalence of psychiatric disorders in children with speech and language disorders. *Journal of the American Academy of Child Psychiatry* 25:528–35.

Beitchman, J. H., Nair, R., Clegg, M., and Patel, P. G. 1986. Prevalence of speech and language disorders in 5-year-old kindergarten children in the Ottawa-Carleton region. *Journal of Speech and Hearing Disorders* 51:98–110.

Beitchman, J. H., Wilson, B., Brownlie, E. B., Walters, H., Inglis, A., and Lancee, W. 1996. Long-term consistency in speech/language profiles: II. Behavioral, emotional, and social outcomes. *Journal of the American Academy of Child and Adolescent Psychiatry* 35:815–25.

Beitchman, J. H., Wilson, B., Brownlie, E. B., Walters, H., and Lancee, W. 1996. Long-term consistency in speech/language profiles: I. Developmental and academic outcomes. *Journal of the American Academy of Child and Adolescent Psychiatry* 35:804–824.

Beitchman, J. H., Wilson, B., Johnson, C. J., Leslie, A., Young, A., Adlaf, E., Escobar, M., and Douglas, L. 2001. Fourteen-year follow-up of speech/language impaired and control children: Psychiatric outcome. *Journal of the American Academy of Child and Adolescent Psychiatry* 40:75–82.

Benasich, A., Curtiss, S., and Tallal, P. 1993. Language, learning, and behavioral disturbances in childhood: A longitudinal perspective. *Journal of the American Academy of Child and Adolescent Psychiatry* 32:585–94.

Blishen, B. R., Carroll, W. K., and Moore, C. 1987. The 1981 socioeconomic index for occupations in Canada. *Canadian Review of Sociology and Anthropology* 24:465–88.

Dunn, L. M., and Dunn, L. M. 1981. *Peabody Picture Vocabulary Test - Revised.* Circle Pines, MN: American Guidance Service.

Felsenfeld, S., Broen, P., and McGue, M. 1992. A 28-year follow-up of adults with a history of moderate phonological disorder: Linguistic and personality results. *Journal of Speech and Hearing Research* 35:1114–25.

Felsenfeld, S., Broen, P., and McGue, M. 1994. A 28-year follow-up of adults with a history of moderate phonological disorder: Educational and occupational results. *Journal of Speech and Hearing Research* 37:1341–53.

Hall, P., and Tomblin, J. B. 1978. A follow-up study of children with articulation and language disorders. *Journal of Speech and Hearing Disorders* 43:227–41.

Hammill, D., Brown, V., Larsen, S., and Wiederholt, J. 1994. *Test of Adolescent/Adult Language 3.* Austin, TX: PRO-ED.

Hunt, K. 1965. Grammatical structure written at three grade levels (Research Report No. 3). Urbana IL: National Council of Teachers of English.

Johnson, C. J., Taback, N., Escobar, M., Wilson, B., and Beitchman, J. H. 1999. Local norming of the Test of Adolescent/Adult Language-3 (TOAL-3) in the Ottawa speech and language study. *Journal of Speech-Language-Hearing Research* 42:761–66.

Johnson, C. J., Beitchman, J. H., Young, A., Escobar, M., Atkinson, L., Wilson, B., Brownlie, E. B., Douglas, L., Taback, N., Lam, I., and Wang, M. 1999. Fourteen-year follow-up of children with and without speech/language impairments: Speech/language stability and outcomes. *Journal of Speech, Language, and Hearing Research* 42:744–60.

Kessler, R. C., McGonagle, K. A., Zhao, S., Nelson, C. B., Hughes, M., Eshleman, S., Wittchen, H.-U., Kendler, K. S. 1994. Lifetime and 12-month prevalence of DSM-III-R psychiatric disorders in the United States: Results from the National Comorbidity Survey. *Archives of General Psychiatry* 51:8–19.

King, R., Jones, C., and Lasky, E. 1982. In retrospect: A fifteen-year follow-up report of speech-language disordered children. *Language, Speech, and Hearing Services in the Schools* 13:24–32.

Lahey, M. 1990. Who shall be called language disordered? Some reflections and one perspective. *Journal of Speech and Hearing Disorders* 55:612–20.

Lewis, B., and Freebairn, L. 1992. Residual effects of preschool phonology disorders in grade school, adolescence, and adulthood. *Journal of Speech and Hearing Research* 35:819–31.

Miller, J. F., and Chapman, R. S. 1997. *Systematic Analysis of Language Transcripts.* Madison, WI: University of Wisconsin.

Newcomer, P. L., and Hammill, D. D. 1977. *Test of Language Development.* Austin, TX: Empiric Press.

Stark, R. E., and Tallal, P. 1981. Selection of children with specific language deficits. *Journal of Speech and Hearing Disorders* 46:114–22.

Stothard, S. E., Snowling, M. J., Bishop, D. V. M., Chipchase, B., and Kaplan, C. A. 1998. Language-impaired preschoolers: A follow-up into adolescence. *Journal of Speech, Language, and Hearing Research* 41:407–418.

Tomblin, J. B., Freese, P., and Records, N. 1992. Diagnosing specific language impairment in adults for the purpose of pedigree analysis. *Journal of Speech and Hearing Research* 35:832–43.

Tomblin, J. B., Records, N. L., Buckwalter, P., Zhang, X., Smith, E., and O'Brien, M. 1997. Prevalence of specific language impairment in kindergarten children. *Journal of Speech, Language, and Hearing Research* 40:1245–60.

Ward, C. L. 1990. Prediction of verbal, performance, and full scale IQs from seven subtests of the WAIS-R. *Journal of Clinical Psychology* 46:436–40.

Wechsler, D. 1981a. *Wechsler Adult Intelligence Scale—Revised.* New York: The Psychological Corporation.

Wechsler, D. 1981b. *Wechsler Preschool and Primary Scale of Intelligence.* New York: The Psychological Corporation.

Wilkinson, G. 1993. *Wide Range Achievement Test—3.* Wilmington, DE: Jastak.

Woodcock, R., and Johnson, M. B. 1989. *Woodcock-Johnson Psychoeducational Battery—Revised.* Allen, TX: DLM Teaching Resources.

Young, A., Beitchman, J. H., Johnson, C. J., Atkinson, L., Escobar, M., Douglas, L., and Wilson, B. 2002. Young adult academic outcomes in a longitudinal sample of speech/language impaired and control children. *Journal of Child Psychology and Psychiatry and Allied Disciplines* 43(5):635–45.

Index

(Page numbers in italics indicate material in figures or tables.)